THE FAT THIEF
TAKE BACK YOUR LIFE

HOW TO BEAT YOUR INNER DRAGON

Shaun J. Melarvie M.D. F.A.C.S.

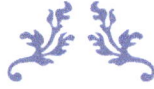

This book is dedicated to the overweight and obese who are ready to change their world. This is for you.

This will be easy to read. It will be quick. You should be able to read it in one or two or three sittings. You could read only the bold type and text boxes and study the pictures and get the primary message; however, the persuasion is within the text, and that is what is needed for you to change your thoughts.

I have built a program for you. It consists of this book or manual, three short, supplemental videos at FatThief.com, tools and reference links at the website as well, and an ongoing online presence and source of support. A support structure is essential in this endeavor of thought and world changing. I will be there for you as much as I can.

This program is presented in a very specific order that will become clear as you progress through the material. I believe that I have taken a common subject and have treated it in an uncommon fashion. I believe you will find it meaningful. I believe I can change your thoughts.

It is all here. The book. The videos. The website. As time goes on, I will publish an e-book version and a supplemental black and white workbook, as well as an audiobook. I will continue to populate FatThief.com with content you will find interesting and helpful on your journey. It is important that you remain engaged.

It is now up to you. I love beginnings, almost as much as good endings. Best wishes.

Shaun Melarvie

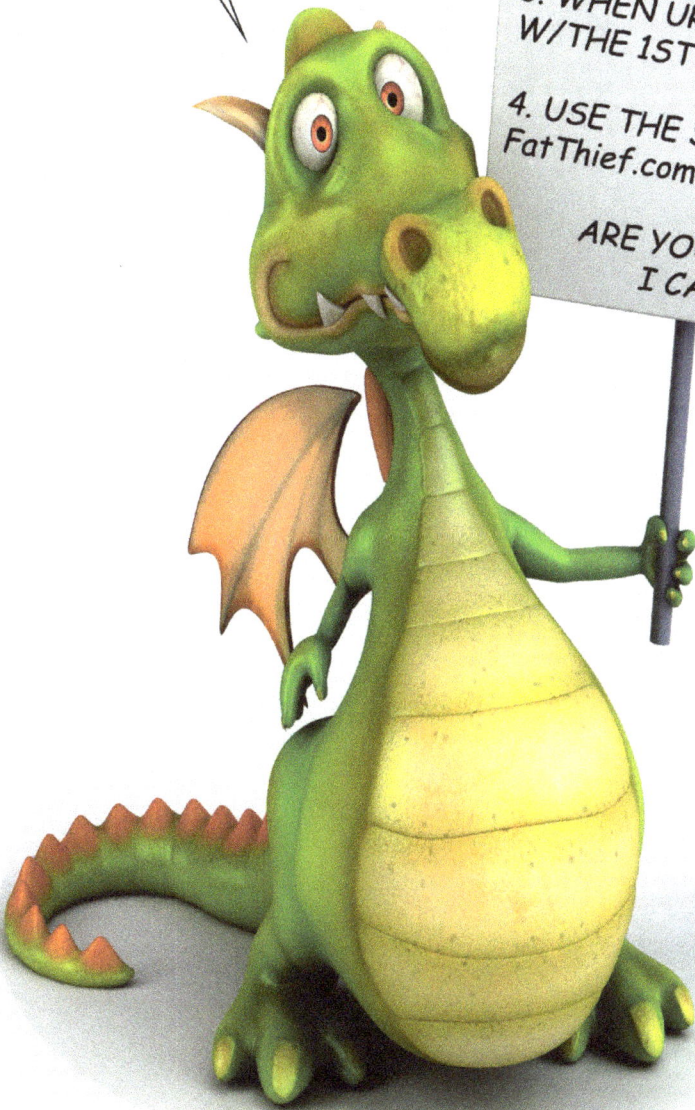

Table of Contents

In the Beginning,

darkness

was upon the

face of the deep.

THESE TEXT BOXES ARE ACTION ITEMS, THINGS YOU SHOULD DO.

YELLOW IS IMPORTANT.

IF IT LOOKS LIKE A CHAINSAW, THAT'S SUPER IMPORTANT. THERE'S ONLY TWO OF THOSE.

These text boxes are informational, typically will emphasize main points and clarifications.

CHAPTER ONE: INTRODUCTION

Why do you want to lose weight? What is your motivator: a wedding, tight clothes, an upcoming appointment with your doctor, a recently disappointing appointment with your doctor, diabetes, a fatty liver, sleep apnea, a heart attack or impending one, a new job, a new boyfriend/girlfriend, Brad Pitt, a beach-body, to get even with someone, just tired of it, don't feel good about yourself, a comment someone made or that you overheard, a break-up, a divorce; or, because you think you're going to die? We all have our reasons. Although any reason is good enough, if it works for you for the rest of your life, which seems to be exceedingly uncommon given the 42% incidence of obesity in middle-aged Americans, I would maintain that the fundamental reason is the last because…

Obesity kills. It is a thief. It steals your life. It may not be as obvious as your heart giving one last whimper, one last squeeze before it gives up pumping your blood through the extra miles of capillaries in all those extra pounds of fat. No, more likely it will be one of the obesity-related illnesses, like diabetes, cardiovascular heart disease, or cancer that does it. It's a "sure thing," like some kind of a technical indicator a day-trader in the stock market might spend a lifetime searching for in order to strike it rich except that in this case it really does come true. Of one thing you may be certain, if you are obese, you will live less, and you will live less well than you would otherwise if you were not.

This is not a conventional diet book. There are already plenty of those. This is a book of how to change your world. The only requirement, the only thing you have to do is this: You must be an active participant in your own reality. You gotta wanna. It's really that simple. You have the power to do this. As Norman Vincent Peale said, "I change my thoughts, I change my world."

I am going to help you change your thoughts. I want to help you change your world. I am going to use three primary arguments. I will be funny. I will be irreverent. I will be reverent. You will laugh. You will think. You will feel. I promise you that. Although my primary focus is on weight control and healthy choices, these arguments and strategies apply to anything that matters.

The structure of this transmission of empowerment will be textual, via an easy to read book of 200 pages with pictures, three short videos, an active online presence and community, and even a personal interaction should you ever be in the same geographical area as I when giving a presentation.

Why me? You might ask. What do I know about any of this stuff? Well, I used to be fat. I know that's a dirty word and is frowned upon; however, obese isn't much better, and especially morbidly obese (that's really bad). The thing is, I never thought of those medical terms when I saw myself in pictures or looked in a mirror. I saw a fat man on a sailboat in pictures from a winter vacation. I saw a fat man staring back at me in the mornings when I was forced to look at myself when getting ready for work, hopeless and despondent, wondering how and exactly when I ever got to that place where I was.

If you're like most people, you or a loved one has suffered a serious illness, a hospitalization, a major surgical procedure. You went to see a doctor, a surgeon. You placed your trust in an individual not personally known to yourself because that person, that individual, had spent a lifetime training and learning how to help you. I am exactly *that* person. If you are obese, I *have been* in that place where you are; I *am in* that place where you wish to be.

I have worked hard my entire life and I have had my passions as I think of them, things that keep me awake at night, things that occupy my mind that I cannot easily turn off. One of my dominant passions is obesity and has been for the past 15 years. I do not know why, other than I have struggled with it most of my adult life. I suppose it is the impossibility of the problem, the challenge, the recidivism (relapse rate), the magnitude, the wide swath it cuts across all demographics, the absolute despair and hopelessness that those so suffering experience on a daily basis--There has to be a better way I cannot help but reason and wonder why.

I feel like my entire life's experiences have led me to this most beautiful intersection with you, the reader, and I would like to express my sincere thanks to you for taking the time to consider these words I have written in my impassioned effort to affect a change in your life, in your world, by causing you to change your thoughts. I will briefly explain the structure of this epistle, which will make it clear that this is not the typical diet book.

I wish to present three primary arguments for you to apply towards your thoughts that might cause you change the way you think. Although these primary arguments would apply to any problem you might be facing, the problem we will be applying them to is obesity.

The reason why my focus is on changing your thoughts is because they are the root cause of the problem facing you, in this case, obesity or being overweight. Anyone can follow a program, do the right things, eat the right foods for a while, but eventually there will be a reversion towards the mean. There always is. It's like the economics of the Dow Jones Industrial Average (DOW). It reverts towards the mean when it extends too far above or below the trendline. It's like a law. It always happens, like an overstretched rubber-band snapping back into place.

Following a diet plan is merely treating the symptom of your dysfunctional thoughts. I say dysfunctional thoughts because if you are obese, it is most likely that your concept of your own body's metabolism is in fact dysfunctional.

It is like using a CPAP machine for sleep apnea or taking anti-hypertensives for hypertension, or insulin for diabetes type 2: you are treating the symptoms of obesity, not in all cases of course, but, in most. You are managing the disease processes, not curing them. It is by addressing the root cause of obesity that you will cure the disease.

> The Root cause of obesity are dysfunctional thoughts relating to your diet; and sometimes dysfunctional thoughts relating to yourself. No diet is going to fix that. You have to fix your thoughts.

Again, it is your thoughts that are the root cause of your obesity, which brings me back to the three arguments I would like to present to you. I think of them as arrows, three arrows that you might place in that imaginary quiver on your back; three arrows, each one stronger than the one that comes before with which you might slay that dragon of obesity, or any other dragon you find before you. They are the arrow of TRUTH, the arrow of REALITY, and the arrow of BELIEF.

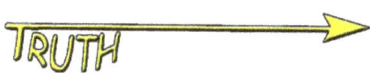

TRUTH ⟶

I believe that if you know the absolute truth about how your body handles energy, you will change your thoughts.

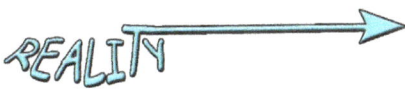

REALITY ⟶

I believe that if you have an understanding of the power you hold to affect your own reality, and a mindful appreciation of your internal thinking, you will empower yourself to make the proper choices and self-select the reality you deserve.

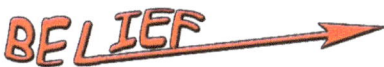

BELIEF ⟶

I believe that if you are able to develop a firm belief in yourself; and, if a spiritual person, able to acknowledge the role of a higher-power, then you will realize an inner strength and grace that will become a shield protecting you from the forces arrayed against you. Although the arrow of belief does imply a spiritual aspect, this is largely individualized and a matter of personal interpretation. It is what you choose to make of it.

Belief is a powerful word, like truth, hope, love, or forgiveness. Belief must begin within. You must believe in yourself, that you can do these things, that you have the power to affect change, that all things are possible; but first you must think them, imagine them, only then may they come true. Although there is a role for faith-based behavioral management strategies, the great majority of the cognitive behavioral strategies I will be addressing are non-spiritual, or secular. The role of belief in a higher power is *in addition to* self-belief and will be addressed, with *additional* behavioral modification strategies, in the last portion of this manual, accessible to those so inclined to pursue it.

This manual will be easily understood. It will be presented succinctly and will not be burdened down by footnotes, references and personal testimonials. All source material not from my head will be referenced in a bibliography or appendix in the back. The only testimonial required is mine. I will start with the truth. I will tell you exactly what to do and how to do it and why you should do it. That might be enough for some; however, for most, it will not be enough because bad habits and bad thoughts die hard, in which case you must continue on because you will need one or both of the remaining arrows.

In the spirit of simplicity and brevity, this is a manual of absolutes, of blacks and whites. There is little nuance. So, buckle up, Buttercup, you've no idea what's coming, but first...

I would like to take this opportunity to introduce you to a cast of characters, two mainly, who will assist in the visual representation of the material I will present. It is my view that the engagement of as many senses as possible will help you better understand; and, if you'll be spending a few hours with me on this journey, we may as well have a little fun *while we walk along*.

When I first had this idea for a combination of prose and visualized text or a graphic-novel-like medium the names of the two primary characters were immediately in my mind, where they were birthed years ago, lying dormant until now. At first, I thought they would be place holders; however, I am so very fond of these two characters that I have known since the first grade that I decided to keep them for they were the gateway to an infinite number of worlds. Let me introduce you to my old friends.

REFER TO THE APPENDICES AT THE END FOR SPECIFIC LISTS TO FOLLOW AND ACTIONS TO COMPLETE. **IT'S ALL THERE.**

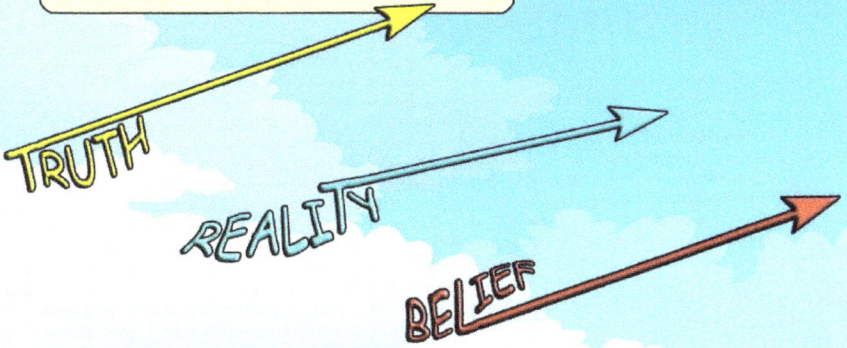

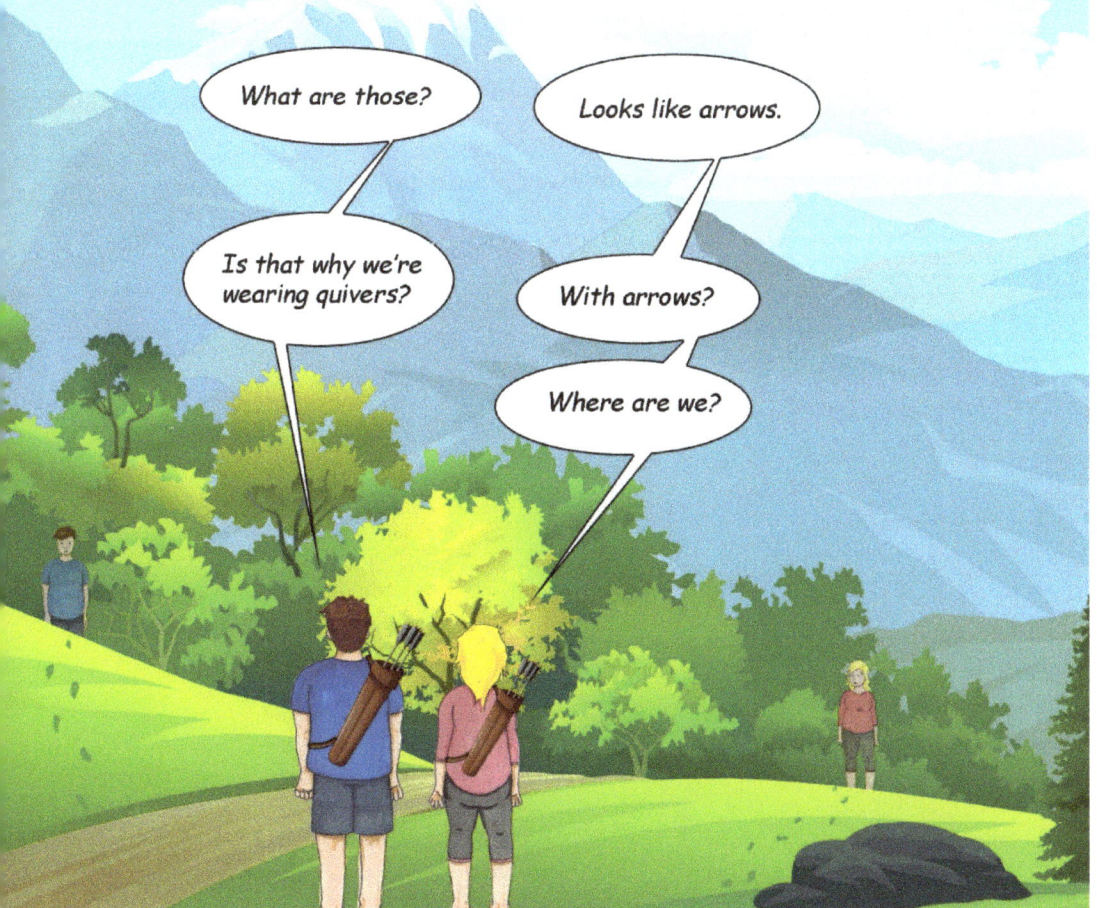

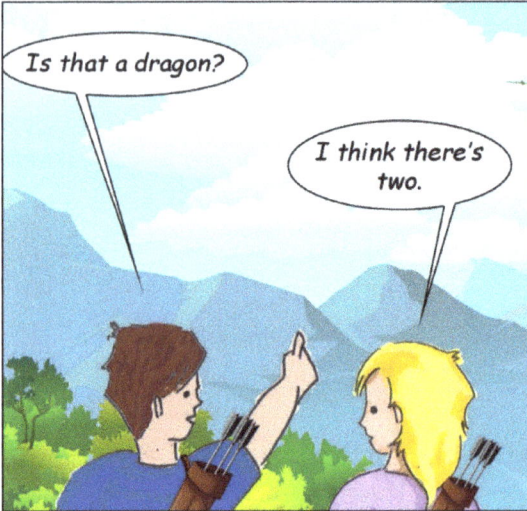

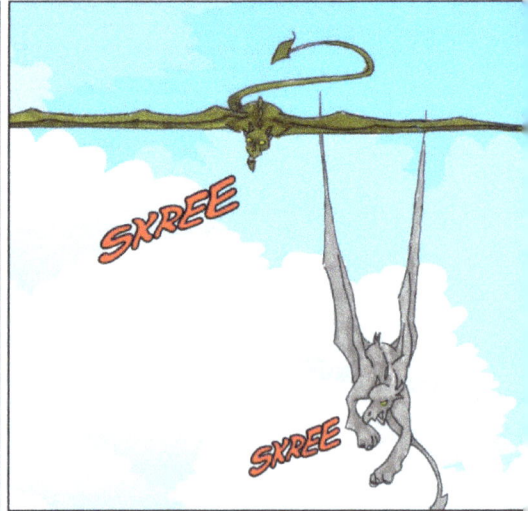

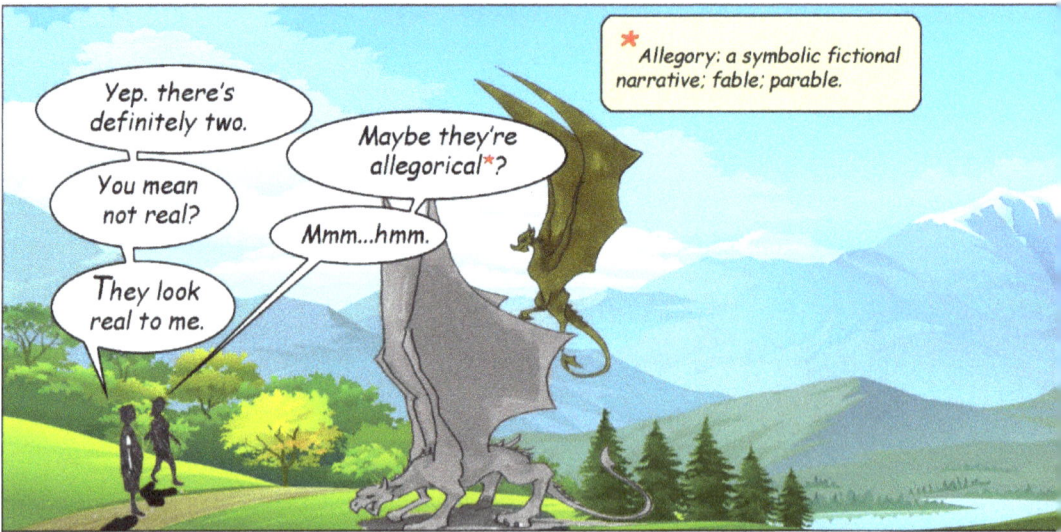

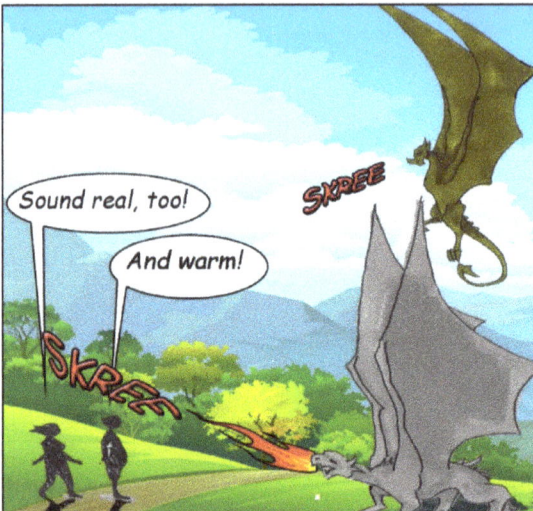

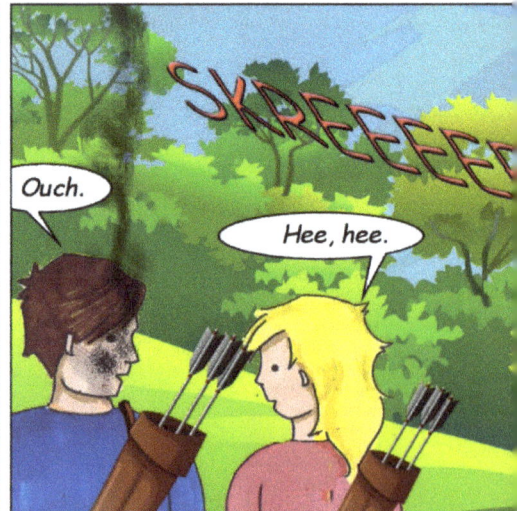

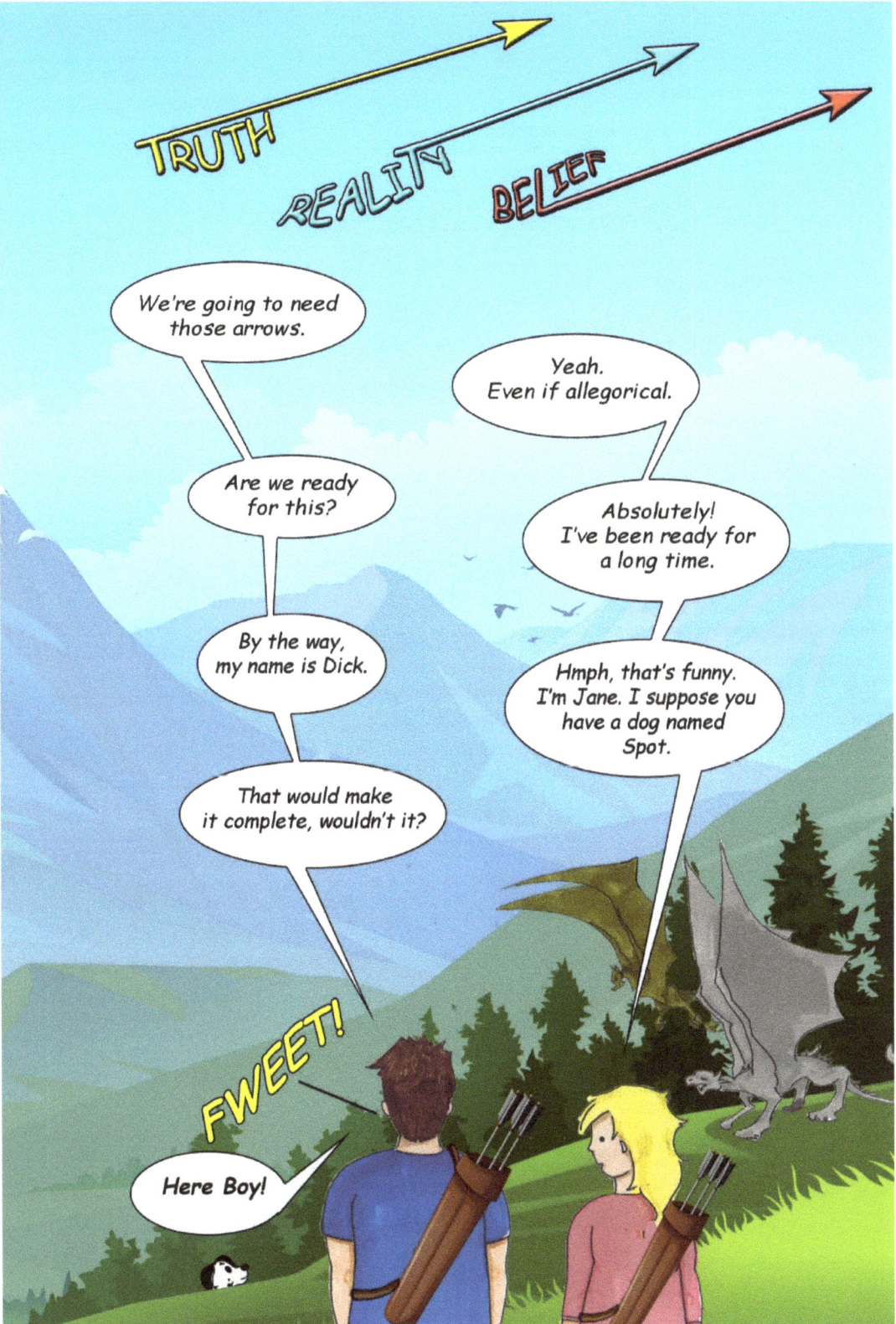

CHAPTER TWO: WHAT IS OBESE?

What is obese? Am I obese?

Hopefully, this should be self-evident. If not, the blunt tool to ascertain obesity is the Body Mass Index (BMI), which is your height divided by your weight for which there are charts and calculators that are widely available. It is an imperfect measure to be sure, but it works well enough for our purposes, and if you can bench-press your weight, boy or girl, more than once, without ruining yourself, you could even give yourself a two or three point "credit." For instance, if you're 5'11" and 220 lbs. you are technically obese, with a BMI of 31. I am 6'3" and used to weigh 300lbs, which means that my BMI was 37. After losing 70 lbs. to 230, my BMI was still a generous 29, just a whisker under the lower end of the obese category at BMI=30; however, I was *big boned*, as they say, and could bench press my body weight a number of times, so I was doing better body-habitus wise than the BMI value would imply.

The important thing is that your own personal BMI serves as a reference point, and unless you are a body builder, values greater than 30 are not desirable. Another reference point to track would be cloth-tape measurements at your neck, chest (nipple level), waist (belly button, or top of hip bone if belly button is below that level, which is bad), and hips (largest part of butt).

So, that's easy. If you're not sure you're obese, check your BMI. If you are not a professional body builder or equivalent, and if your BMI is greater than 30, you are obese. If you want to change your thoughts and thereby change your world, then, measure yourself at the four levels, as above, write down the values in the first appendix at the end of this book, or in a diary or in a digital spreadsheet or tracking app on your phone; and, keep reading.

Body Mass Index

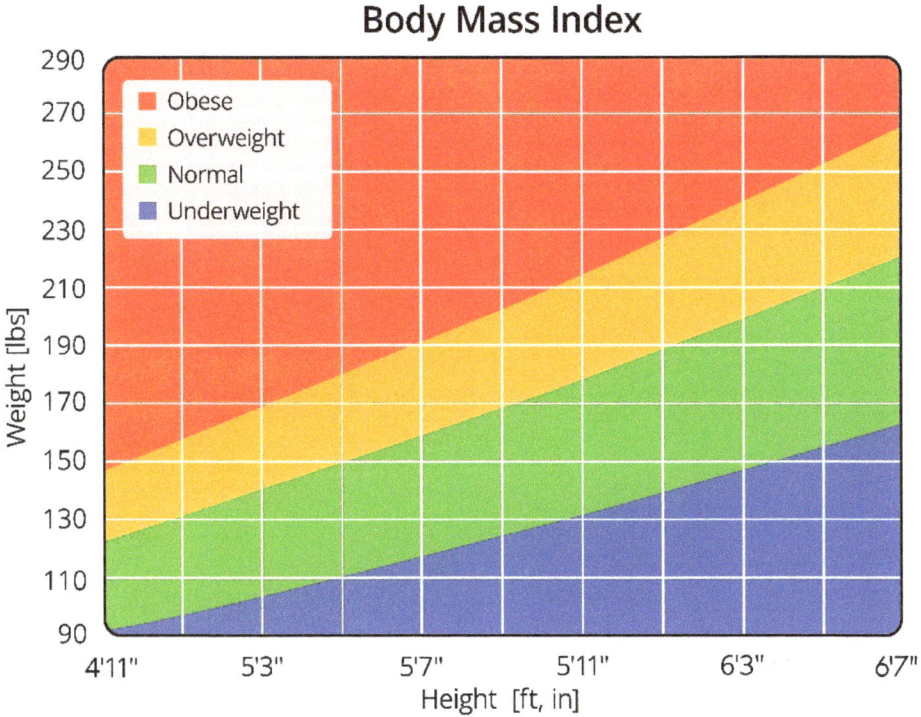

The next 100 pages are the most important because they represent the truth, relative to obesity, which is our First Arrow. You need that. You need to know the argument of the truth, specific to obesity, in order to use the remaining two arrows. I have divided the argument into **four phases** that are designed to be completed in that order, and the completion of each phase will result in a positive effect relative to your weight. The further along you advance in the phases, the more weight you will lose. These first four phases represent the arrow of truth. You must complete the arrow of truth. It is primary.

Phase I: The Diet
Phase II: Energy
Phase III: Insulin, Metabolism, Death
Phase IV: Exercise, Loose Ends

I finish the four phases with some loose ends that don't fit neatly into the phases, as illustrated, before moving on to the second arrow. If you wanted, you could read these first 100 pages (with lots of pictures) and get started at any step along the way. Technically, you wouldn't need to complete the manual; BUT, the risk of recidivism (gaining weight back after losing it) is significant, which is the purpose of the last two arrows, the arrow of reality and the arrow of belief. If you are reading this manual, you need help. Let me help you.

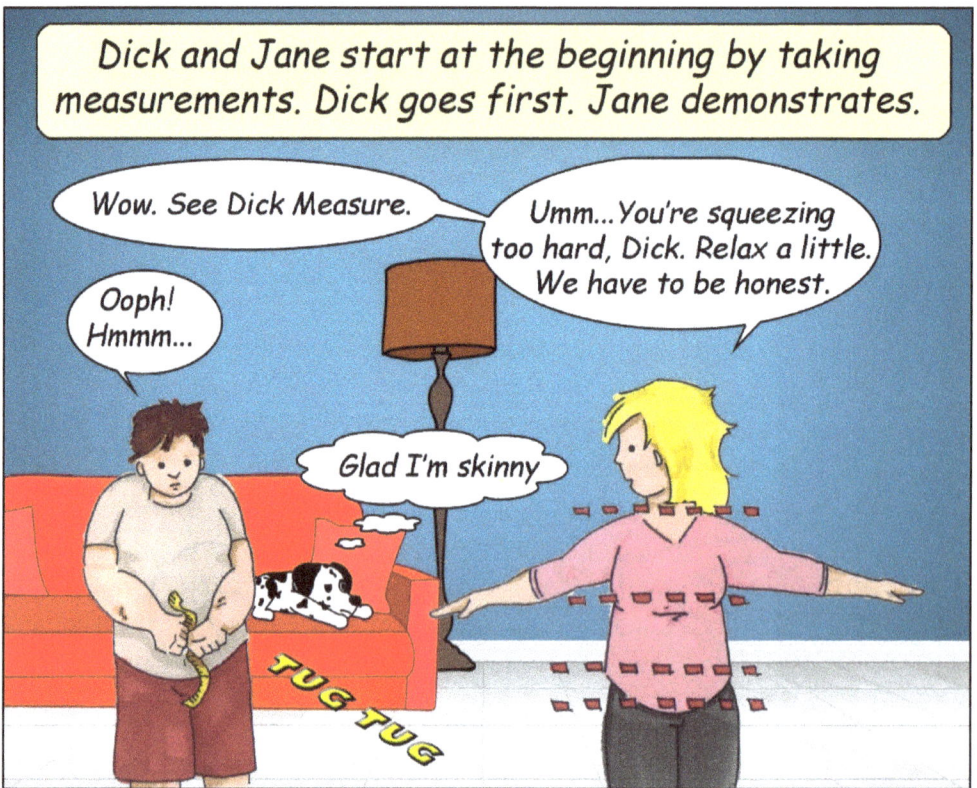

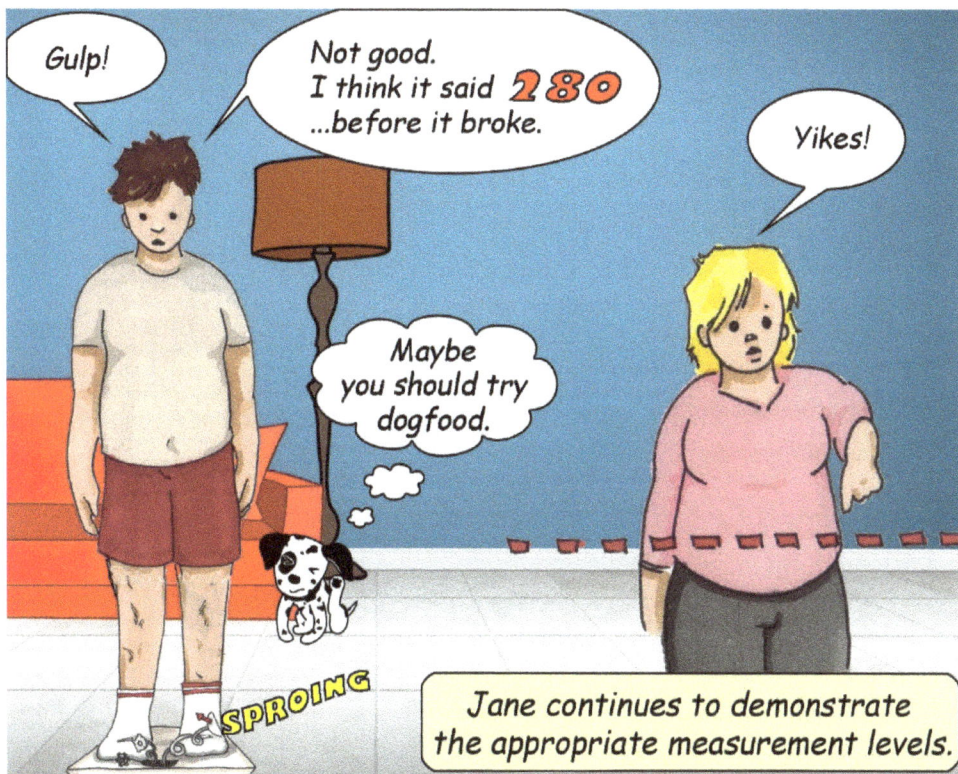

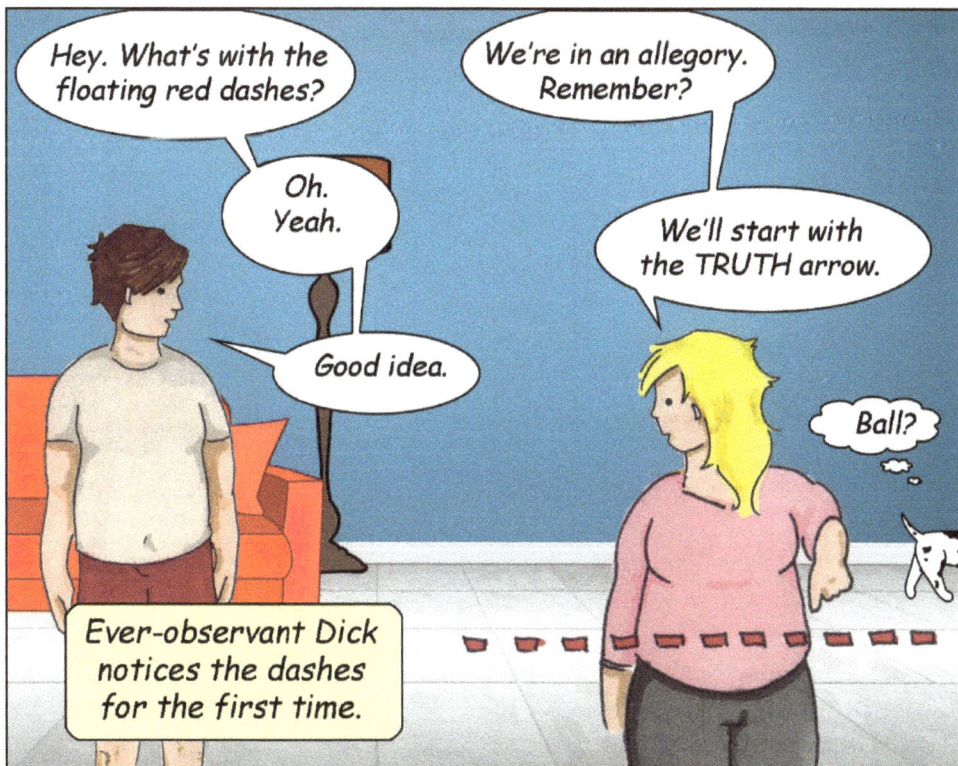

CHAPTER THREE: Phase I: THE DIET

Phase I:
1. **Pick your diet.**
2. Prepare your home.
3. Have a strategy for eating away from home.

What diet should I follow? Is there one that's the best?

There are two competing themes in the diet-universe, let's call it the *dietverse*. It is not an exhaustive list, but you will get the idea.

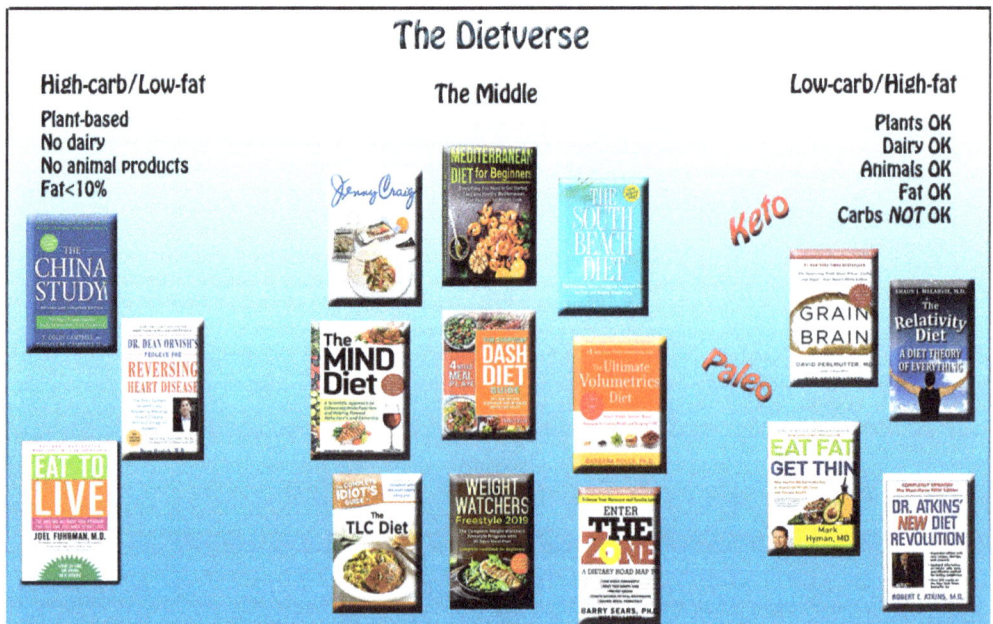

All diets fit somewhere within this spectrum. In the diagram, on the far left, are listed some diet models that represent of the first of these competing themes; the plant-based diets.

Most of these diets exclude or sharply limit the intake of animal products, including dairy. With this limitation of animal protein and the weight assigned to plant-based foods, these diets are generally higher-carb/lower-fat strategies. Some of the proponents of these diets suggest that a fat intake of over 10% of your daily caloric needs is bad, and that meat and eggs are harmful.

The second competing theme, on the right in the illustration, is pretty much the opposite, as would be expected with extremes. These diets are the popular low-carb, ketogenic diets that do not discourage the ingestion of animal products, but they do sharply limit carbohydrate intake to less than 50 grams a day, which is roughly equivalent to two slices of bread. There is no limit on plant-based foods other than the carbohydrate content; therefore, most fruit is discouraged as it is high in sugar, even if organic and completely natural. For instance, one cup of cherries has twenty grams of carbohydrates. Have you ever eaten just one cup of cherries? Ever? *I didn't think so.*

Although dairy is not specifically excluded, the same consideration is given to the carbohydrate content. Generally, dairy is more forgiving, relative to carbohydrates, than fruit. Watch out for added sugar in yogurt, or in anything else for that matter.

Because of the sharp limitation in carbohydrates, and since the calories have to come from somewhere, these diets are by default low-carb/higher-fat, higher-protein strategies. The proponents of these diets don't particularly care what you eat, as long as the total carbohydrate intake is limited. I understand that this is a gross simplification, but this is a book of absolutes for the purposes of brevity and clarity.

So. These are the extremes: high-carb/low-fat, plant-based, no animal products versus low-carb/whatever the hell you want, as long as it's low-carb. I've read several authors making these respective arguments, and I must admit that there is a slight whiff of religion relative to their arguments; however, I'd have to say that the religious whiff is stronger on the left with the plant-based diets than it is with the low-carb diets. I don't want to waste any time on the ideology of either approach. The pertinent books making the respective arguments are demonstrated in the illustration for your reference. We've more important things to focus on here.

THERE ARE THREE BASIC DIET PHILOSOPHIES TO CHOOSE FROM:
1. PLANT-BASED, HIGHER-CARB/LOW FAT
2. LOW-CARB/HIGHER FAT
3. CALORIC RESTRICTION W/O SPECIFIC CARB OR FAT RESTRICTIONS.

PICK THE STRATEGY YOU PREFER.

As with everything, between two extremes there is a middle, and typically the middle is larger than either extreme. This too, is reflected in the diagram. Because the two extremes are so restrictive, they are, by default, largely caloric limiting. What I mean by this is that counting calories is not as crucial at the extremes as it is with the diets in the larger middle where there is the *combination of* carbohydrates and fat, which is where folks get in trouble. It is the *combination of* fat and carbohydrate that kills, and especially the combination of sugar and refined carbohydrates and the "bad" fats: --they'll kill you for sure.

Therefore, for all the diets in the middle, where there is the combination of significant carbohydrate intake, over 100 grams per day, and fat, it is more important to count calories. In truth, given our baseline human condition and an inherent difficulty with boundaries and limits, for many, counting calories in all cases is a good idea, at least until you have a firm grasp of what a calorie represents as it relates to portion size, because in many cases the victim of the dragon of obesity has a distorted view of proper portion sizes.

One Portion. Honest.

The combination of **CARBOHYDRATES** and **FAT** in excess is a recipe for disaster.

You need to sharply **limit** FAT or CARBOHYDRATES; **or** limit them both more **moderately** (a diet "in the middle").

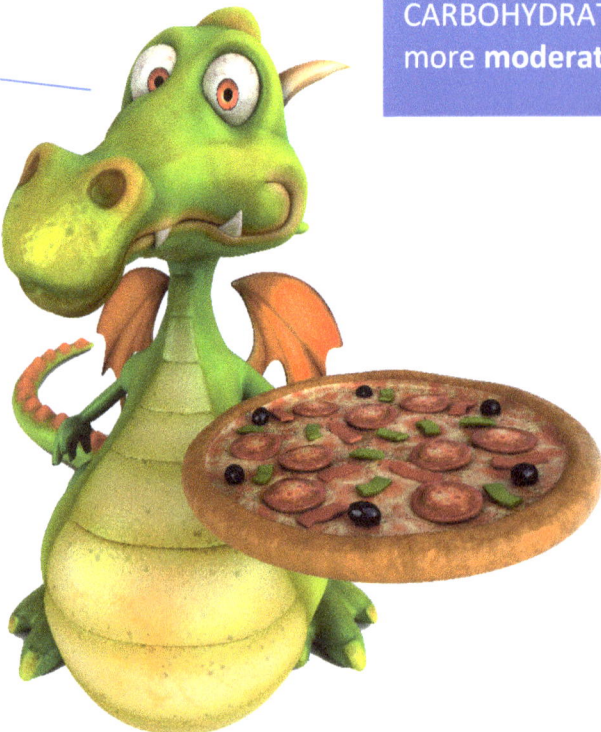

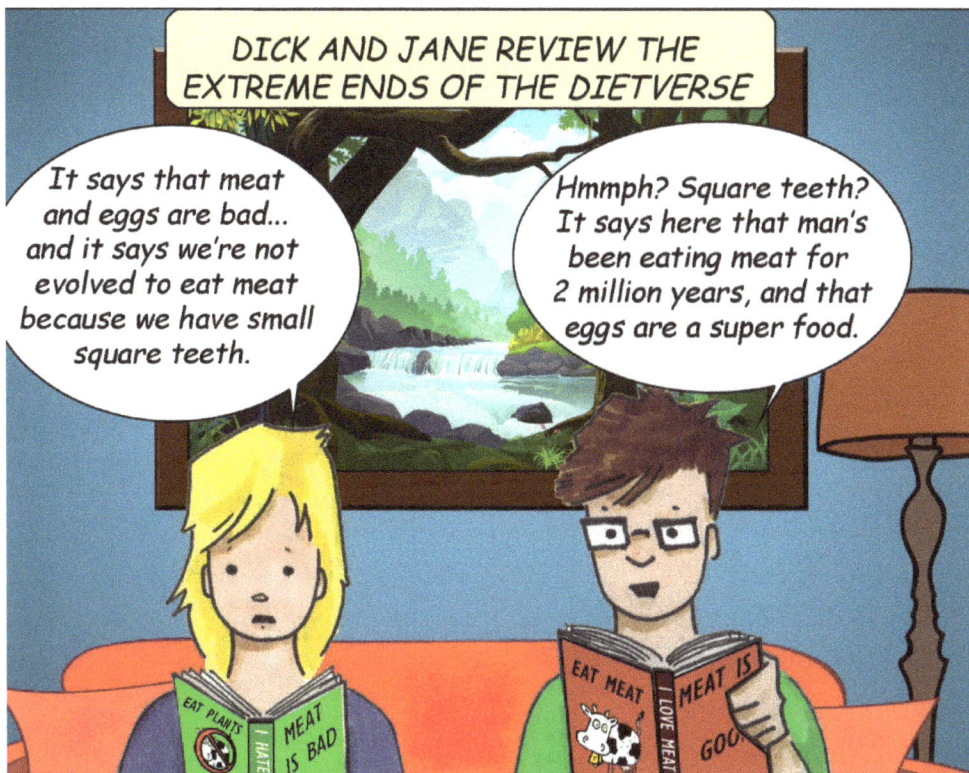

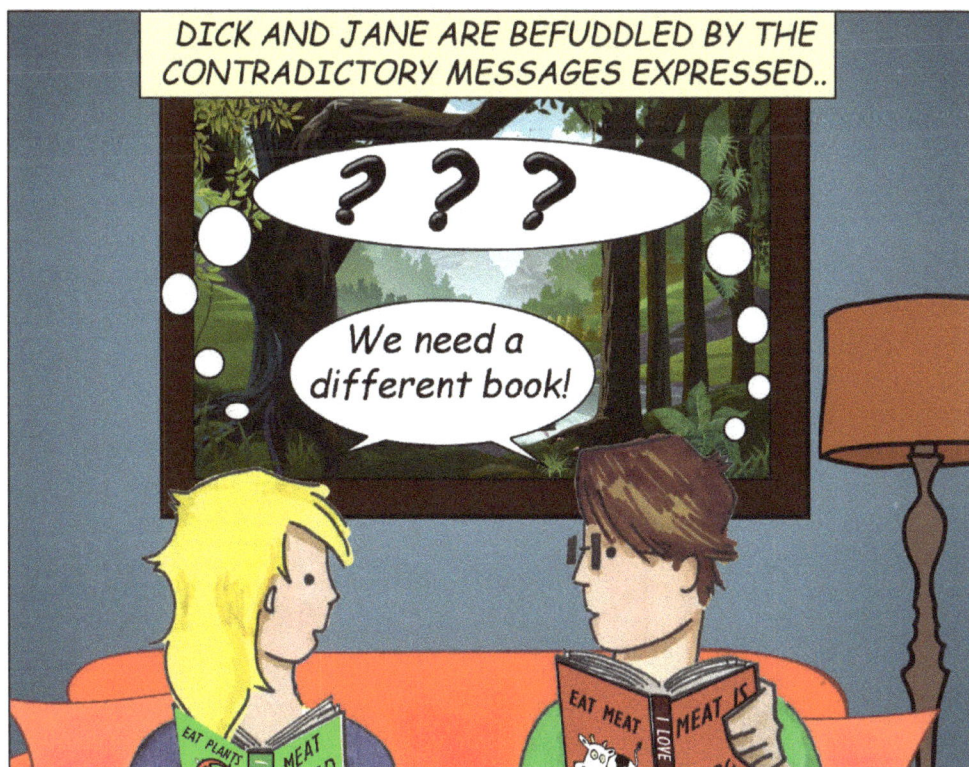

So? What diet should I follow? Is one diet better than the rest?

Pick whatever one you like. They all work, if you can follow them, which is of course the rub. Most people can follow a diet for a while, but…

If you were to read all these books, you would find a common thread that runs through every one of them. The gross commonality is that they ALL discourage the ingestion of sugar (not of whole foods), refined carbohydrates (white bread) and the bad fats (fast food, chips, frosting, cake, pie, grain-fed, fatty meat). *The only outlier is the traditional Atkins, which did not distinguish bad fat from good fat.* If all you were to do were to cut out these things, then you would most likely lose weight and could stop reading, but I'm hoping you won't because I'm just getting started.

THINGS ALL DIETS HAVE IN COMMON *(with examples)*

1. NO SUGAR: CANDY, SWEETS, SODA, POWDERED DONUTS
2. NO REFINED CARBOHYDRATES: WHITE BREAD, PASTA, RICE
3. NO BAD FATS: FAST FOOD, CHIPS, FROSTING, FRIES

If eating meat is against your religion, then pick a plant-based diet, and keep reading. If you don't have any specific dietary restrictions, pick whichever diet is closest to how you might like to eat for the rest of your life, and you don't need the specific diet-book, you mainly need the recipe book that lists the foods and meal plans for whichever diet it is you're interested in.

BUY A COOKBOOK OF THE DIET YOU PICK, WITH FAST AND EASY RECIPIES.

It is important that you look through the books first, so I'd go to a bookstore, because you have to make sure that the meals and ingredients are something that you recognize, actually could make, and actually would make. For instance, if a recipe calls for braised daikon or ikan bilis, I'd avoid that book; or, if a recipe lists castoreum, I'd definitely not buy that one as castoreum is a secretion from the anal glands of beavers; or, if a typical meal preparation time is two hours and thirty minutes, pick another. Fast and easy; that's what you want.

If you're not quite sure and are on the fence, pick the Mediterranean Diet plan. It finishes towards the top of popular diets year after year. It is as much in the middle as you can get, and you can cheat to either side, insofar as plant-based/animal-product avoidance versus low-carb/animals and dairy OK.

Ketogenic diets are already similar to the Mediterranean Diet in that they are higher good-fat; the difference is that they are low-carb, including a very limited intake of grain, fruit, and complex carbs such as corn and starchy vegetables.

> *In 2019 U.S. News and World Report ranked the Mediterranean Diet as BEST overall. The DASH diet was #2. The Mediterranean diet consistently finishes in the top of the lists year after year.*

As for myself, I am biased towards the ketogenic side of things. A bone-in-ribeye is definitely not against my religion, and lower-carb diets have always worked easier for me, and lastly, as you will see, I think they make more sense metabolically.

Lastly, I should mention two other diets that don't neatly fit into the diagram previously displayed. The first of these is Intermittent Fasting for which there is a strong metabolic argument that makes sense to me and I will spend more time on this before we're done. The second strategy is the Mindful Diet, or variations thereof, in which there are no specific restrictions other than common sense (fudge, greasy burgers, potato-chips bad/celery good) and the primary focus is on behavioral modification and eating what seems right and until you are full and so on and so forth.

Relative to the so-called mindful eating, I don't see it as having a significant role on the front end as I think that the obese individual, as I once was, needs to first learn how to eat mindfully; however, the behavioral modification aspects have utility early on and I have some strong feelings and powerful thoughts in that regard. Afterall, they are a significant component of my arrows, my three specific strategies to slay the dragon.

BIAS ALERT

I HAVE A BIAS TOWARDS A LOW CARB DIET, OF LESS THAN 150 CARBS/DAY. A **KETOGENIC DIET** IMPLIES A CARBOHYDRATE INTAKE OF <50 GRAMS/DAY, WHICH IS MORE AGGRESSIVE AND MAY REQUIRE MEDICAL SUPERVISION IF ON MEDICATIONS.

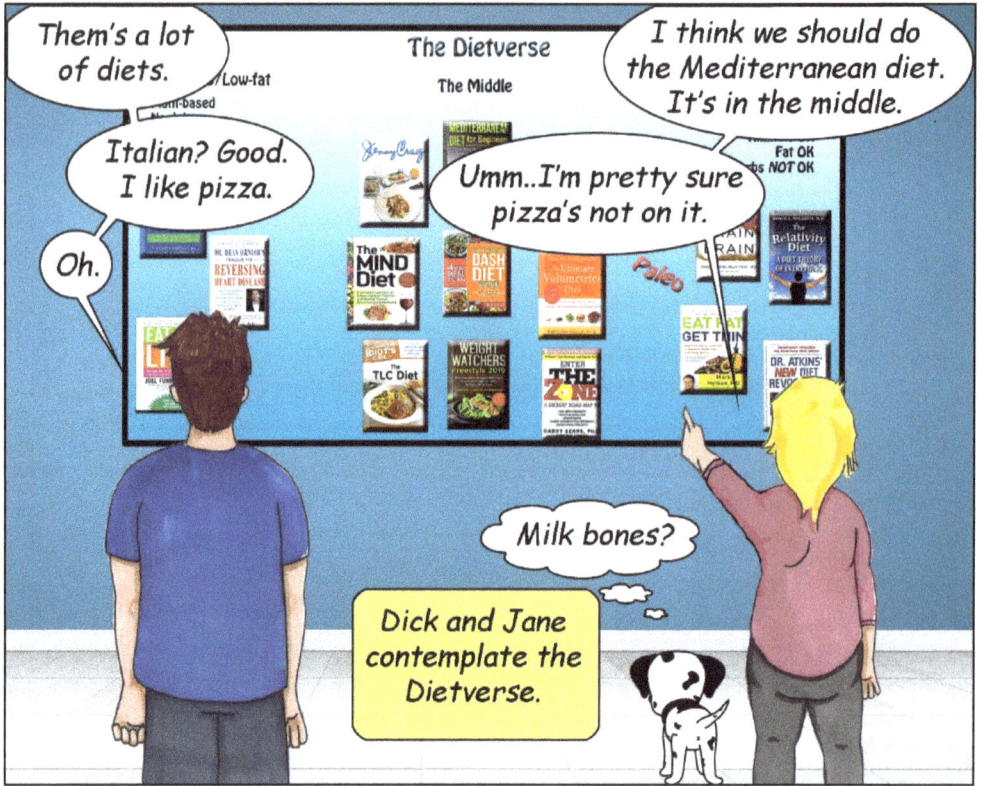

Dick and Jane contemplate the Dietverse.

Phase I:
1. Pick your diet.
2. **Prepare your home.**
3. Have a strategy for eating away from home.

Great. I've got a couple of books. What do I do now?

Now, you must fortify your castle. You must prepare your home. Your home is your safe place and you must build a moat and other barriers to keep out the dragon. The most important barriers will be the mental ones that we will be addressing, which are the primary focus of this manual, but there is one very easy and obvious physical fortification that you now must do.

Establish your safe places. Your home is primary, but you should add your car, and place of employment to the list. You must remove all foods of the devil from these places for they are the bait with which the dragon will slay you.

> Your home is your safe place. So, **make It safe**.

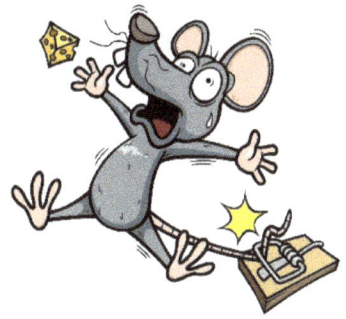

Like the slice of cheddar on the coiled spring that slays the mouse, so too will the poisonous sugar, refined carbohydrates and bad fats slay you. Eventually.

Non-dairy creamer (trans-fat): Gone. Chips and Ritz (trans-fat, refined carbs): Gone. Cookies, cake, ice-cream (sugar, bad-fat, refined carbs): Gone. Hard candies in the center console: Gone. You get the drift. If you don't know, read the label; if it's bad: Gone. A general rule is that if there are too many degrees of separation from what came out of the ground or off the butcher block, it's probably bad. In general, it should look like something that was grown or recently killed for it to be safe. Organic is better than not, such as free-range poultry and eggs; and grass-fed meat is better than commercial, grain-fed meat.

Once you remove all the bait of the dragon you may be wondering what's left. I mean *I get the part about eating healthy meals, but what about the in-between times?* For all but the most ascetic of folks, those monk-like creatures to which self-mortification might come naturally, we needs some options, like Gollum needs the ring. These foods can be anything, as long as you follow the rules; no sugar, no refined carbs, no bad fats. What works for you? For me, I've found that I might make a protein shake with blueberries. I like olives, pickled herring, pickled turkey gizzards, sardines, cottage cheese, yogurt, high-fiber multi-grain crackers with a nut spread (limiting the crackers to one serving). Raw vegetables work, but I don't have them often. Pickled artichokes are good, plain pickles too. The important thing is that if you eat good meals, there is really no need to eat much in between meals. There is no benefit to eating every two to three to four hours. We'll talk more of this later.

Along those same lines: Any candy, gum, junk-food in your car or at work: Gone. Work is kind of a special place because you cannot make that a safe place, unless you are the boss because colleagues, often victims of the dragon themselves, will bring their bait to work to share with you. This can be hard, especially if you are in the intermittent fasting mode and didn't have breakfast and its break-time around 10 AM and there's a chance you might be ravenous and weak of heart. *What're you going to do?* I don't know what will work for you, to be honest, because each work environment is different. One option, if you're not the boss, is to let your fellow comrades know that you are dieting and to not be offended if you decline the offerings of their bait, or if you take your break in another area, away from the odors and site of the aforementioned bait. If you're the boss, that's easy. You might simply say something like, "Sorry, proletarians, bringing bait is not allowed as it may be perceived as threatening to a fellow comrade's sense of well-being."

PLEASE REFER TO APPENDIX B:
HOW TO PREPARE YOUR CASTLE.

Phase I:

1. Pick your diet.
2. Prepare your home.
3. **Have a strategy for eating away from home.**

Now that I've fortified my castle and other safe places, what do I do if I'm not in a safe place?

This pretty much means, *what do I do if I eat out?* which is a lot easier than it used to be thanks to market forces, but it still requires a slight strain of self-denial, especially if you eat out more than once a week. My wife and I eat out once-a-week and when they bring the bread by, and if it's wheat, we tear into it like there's no tomorrow, usually a 60/40 split. Guess who comes out on top? It's not the pretty one.

By now, it should be obvious what you should and shouldn't eat and roughly how much, so if you're eating out of the home you must pick a restaurant that has good choices, and most of them do. No pasta, salad instead of soup, oil and vinegar is better than dressing, a protein entrée, preferably without breading, and vegetables. If the starch selection includes a sweet potato or wild rice, choose that over a white potato or fries, or just have extra vegetables. If you do get a salad dressing, avoid the low-fat ones because that means high-fructose corn syrup, and that means poison, basically.

Obviously, as at home, you must not expose yourself to the food of the devil. It is simple enough to say *NO* to a plastic, table-top, food-spattered, well-fingered flipchart of desserts; however, saying *NO* to the dragon who brings by the freshly baked bait tray is a more difficult matter. Tell your server as you order that you are not interested in the dessert tray if they have one.

You now know enough to get started. If you are morbidly obese, you are currently far away from the place that phase one represents, and simply picking your diet will begin yielding success, but that is only the beginning because the most important part is *changing your thoughts* so that you can do this for the rest of your long, well-lived life--that is my goal for you.

If you are less obese or just overweight and want to lose 20-40 pounds but seem to be stuck on a plateau, you'll need to keep reading. There is much more you can and should do. We haven't even gotten to the arrows yet. I almost feel sorry for the dragon.

> PLEASE REFER TO APPENDIX C:
> *HOW TO EAT OUTSIDE THE WALL.*

In Summary

1. PICK A DIET PLAN: MY BIAS IS TOWARDS A LOW-CARB KETOGENIC, ANTI-INFLAMMATORY STRATEGY. IT IS MY FEELING THAT THESE DIETS ARE EASIER TO COMPLY WITH AS THEY ARE LESS RESTRICTIVE THAN THE PLANT-BASED, ANIMAL-PRODUCT-AVOIDANCE STRATEGY; BUT, YOU'RE THE BOSS. PICK WHATEVER YOU WANT.
2. PREPARE YOUR CASTLE: MAKE YOUR HOME A SAFE PLACE. IT IS YOUR FORTRESS OF SOLITUDE THAT SHOULD BE IMPERVIOUS TO THE DRAGON. HAVE A STRATEGY FOR HOW YOU'RE GOING TO EAT WHEN OUTSIDE THE WALL.

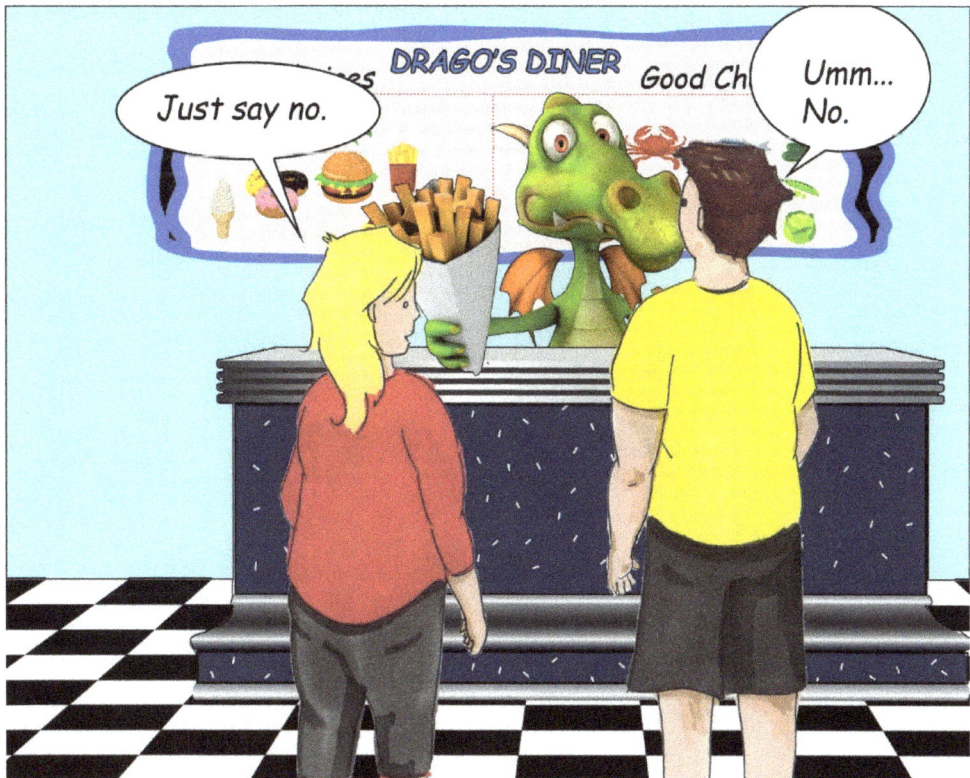

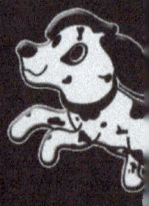

CHAPTER FOUR: Phase II: energy

Phase II:

1. **Understand the truth of a calorie.**
2. Establish your daily caloric need for a weight-loss of 1-2lbs./week.
3. Be Accountable. Be Honest.
4. Get started by controlling the calories IN.

Phases II, III, and IV represent the arrow of truth. If you can wrap your mind around the reality of human metabolism and obesity, *then you will know the truth, and the truth will set you free*. I must confess that the prior two independent clauses are from John 8:32 in which the truth represented God, and the freedom represented freedom from any worldly impediments such as sin, misery or ignorance; all three being, to some extent, components of obesity, if you think about it. Gluttony is one of the seven deadly sins, and I found that the more obese I was, the more miserable I was. I was too ignorant for too long about too many things too important to be ignorant of.

What exactly does a calorie mean and how will knowing that make a difference?

A really cool way to think about this is to recognize that we are all imperfect carbon-based bomb-calorimeters whose primary purpose is to burn energy. *And, pray tell, what is a bomb-calorimeter?*

A bomb calorimeter is a simple apparatus that consists of a small steel chamber placed inside of a larger insulated chamber that is filled with a known quantity of water. Both chambers are sealed, and the inner chamber contains a sample of fuel, for instance, 1 gram of fat, and for the sake of simplicity let us say that the amount of water is exactly 1 kilogram. Of course, the apparatus has thermometers and electrodes and very exact ways to measure things. When the electrode is activated, the fuel sample burns completely away and the energy generated is all in heat, and it raises the temperature of the water by some amount.

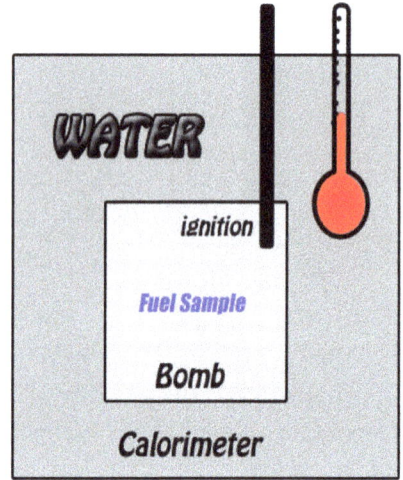

WATER

ignition

Fuel Sample

Bomb

Calorimeter

One calorie equals the amount of energy it takes to raise one gram of water one degree Celsius (same as Centigrade).

The definition of calorie, small "**c**", is the amount of energy it takes to raise the temperature of 1 gram of water 1 degree Celsius. Since this is a very small unit of measure, the more commonly used unit is the kilocalorie or large "**C**", which is 1000 calories (small "c").

A Food Calorie, big "C" (what you see on the label) equals 1 kilocalorie, which is 1000 calories, small "c".

Food calories are always kilocalories (big "C") even if listed as a small "c".

So, logically, a **C**alorie (1000 calories) is the amount of energy it takes to raise the temperature of 1 kilogram (1000 grams) of water 1 degree Celsius.

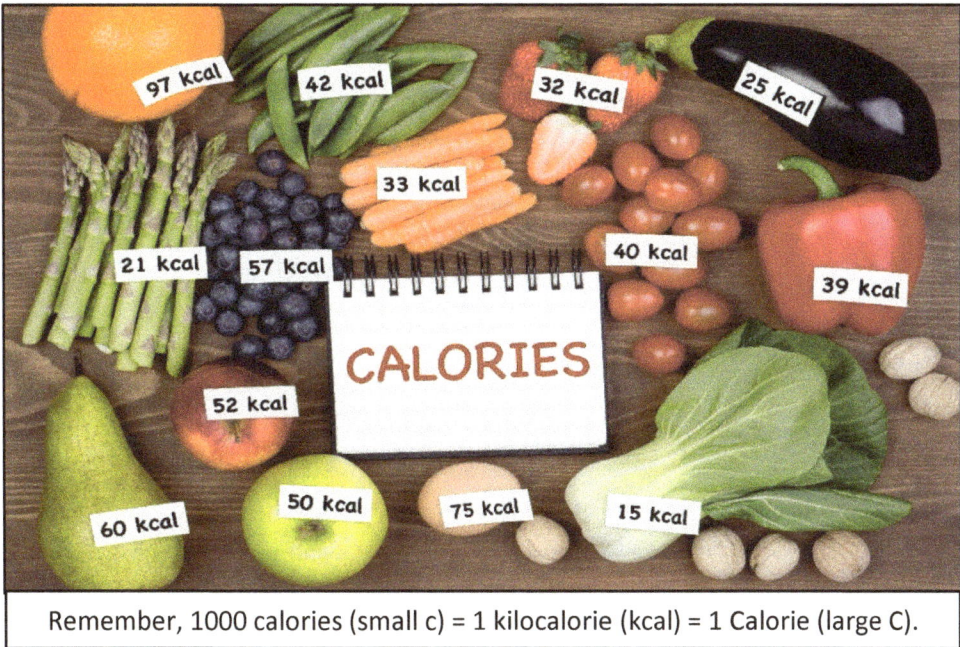

Remember, 1000 calories (small c) = 1 kilocalorie (kcal) = 1 Calorie (large C).

Therefore, with the combustion of our 1 gram of fat in the bomb calorimeter, the temperature of the 1 kilogram of water will rise nine degrees Celsius because the one gram of fat contains nine **C**alories (kilocalories) of energy. This is simply a representation of a universal law, **the first law of thermodynamics**, the law of the conservation of energy, which states that energy can neither be created nor destroyed. In this case, exactly 9 Calories of energy contained in fat is converted to exactly 9 Calories of heat (energy). As a bomb calorimeter, even if imperfect, if you consume energy, you burn it and if you don't burn it you store it for another day, and you know what that means.

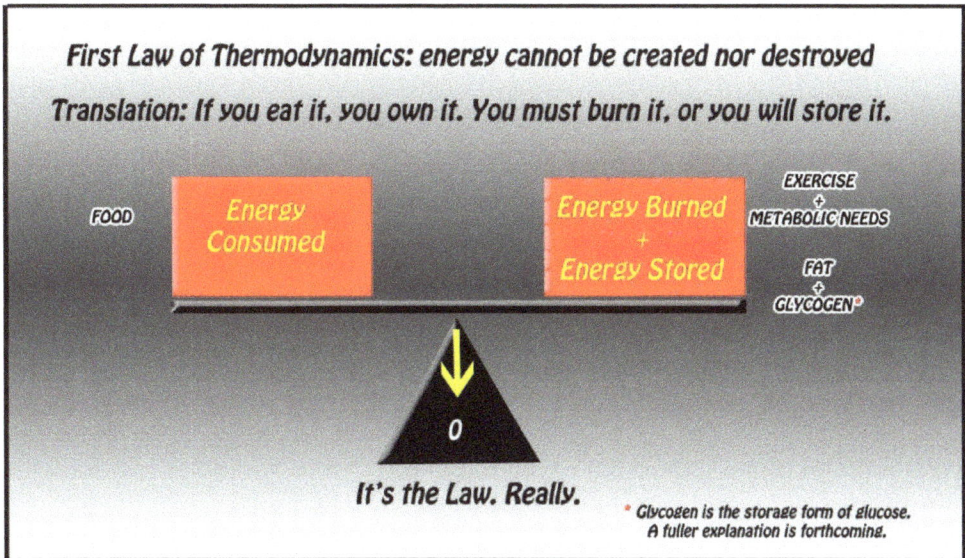

First Law of Thermodynamics: energy cannot be created nor destroyed

Translation: If you eat it, you own it. You must burn it, or you will store it.

FOOD → **Energy Consumed**

Energy Burned + Energy Stored → EXERCISE + METABOLIC NEEDS; FAT + GLYCOGEN*

0

It's the Law. Really.

* Glycogen is the storage form of glucose. A fuller explanation is forthcoming.

Now, if you put a sugar cube containing 5 grams of glucose (sugar) in a bomb calorimeter; and place a cube of sweet potato containing 5 grams of glucose in another bomb calorimeter; both of them will yield exactly 20 Calories because one gram of carbohydrate/sugar holds four Calories of energy (4x5=20). Both forms of energy in the bomb calorimeter yield the same result. *As an imperfect bomb calorimeter, do you think that both forms of energy yield the same result in yourself?*

Consider six pumps of liquid butter *(saturated+trans-fat)* at the theater over a giant bucket of popcorn: If you isolated 5 of the roughly 100 grams of fat from it and placed it in the bomb calorimeter; then placed 5 grams of olive oil in another bomb calorimeter; both of them would yield 45 Calories of energy because one gram of fat holds nine Calories (5x9=45).

Both samples yield the same result. *As an imperfect, carbon-based bomb calorimeter, do you think both types of fat would yield the same result in yourself?*

> Industrial trans-fats are vegetable oils that are altered to make them solid at room temperatures.
>
> They are found in fried foods, baked goods, frozen pizza, cookies.
>
> Trans-fats increase your bad cholesterol, LDL.

There has long been a belief that a change in weight was a simple calculation of calories in versus calories out, and that the calories were the only thing that mattered, as if you were a simple, perfect bomb calorimeter. According to this way of thinking, as long as you controlled the equation of calories in minus calories out, then the calculated change in weight would occur with the given that 3,500 calories equals one pound of fat. Simple. Easy. **Wrong**.

I believe that the idea of *calories in equals calories out* is somewhat true; however, over the past many years there has been much writing on good calories and bad calories and bad fats and good fats, and that is all true too. In fact, it is more true and more applicable than the simple *calories-in equals calories-out* proposition. The bad calories, and by that I mean to say sugar and refined carbohydrates, and the bad fats certainly have negative implications relative to their impact on our metabolism and by their stimulation of an unhealthy pro-inflammatory state, which leads to a whole host of problems that are life-altering and life-limiting.

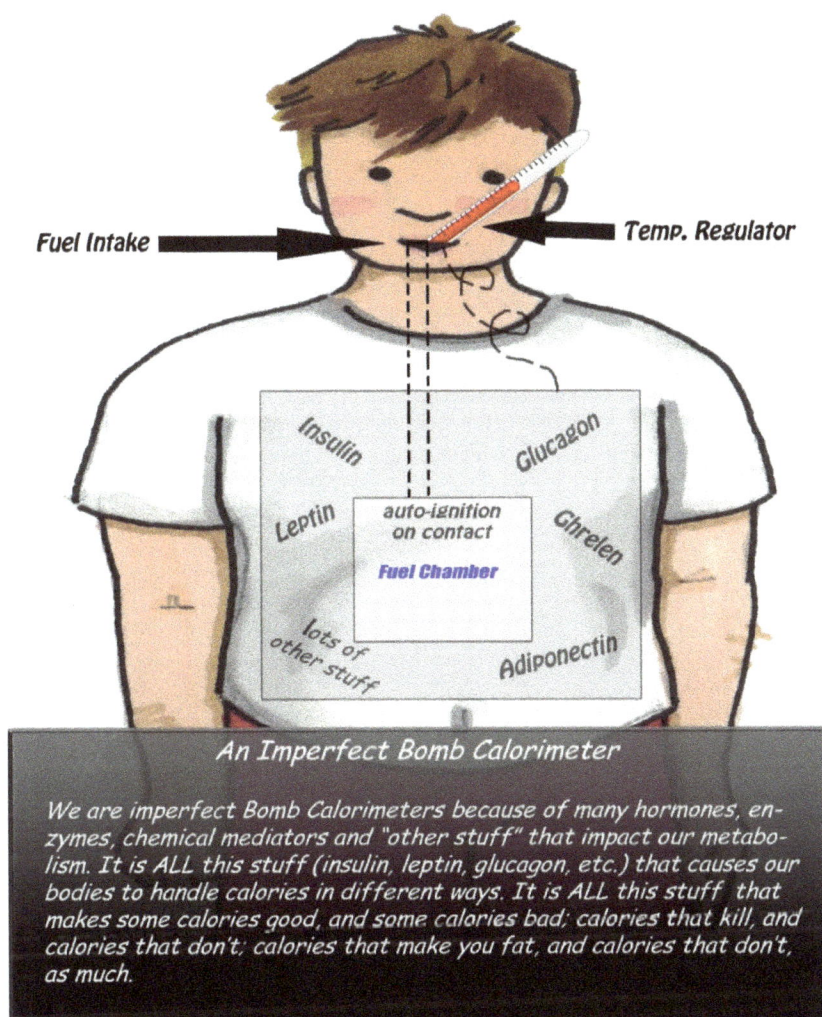

An Imperfect Bomb Calorimeter

We are imperfect Bomb Calorimeters because of many hormones, enzymes, chemical mediators and "other stuff" that impact our metabolism. It is ALL this stuff (insulin, leptin, glucagon, etc.) that causes our bodies to handle calories in different ways. It is ALL this stuff that makes some calories good, and some calories bad: calories that kill, and calories that don't; calories that make you fat, and calories that don't, as much.

The energy placed in your own carbon-based bomb calorimeter does still count, whether it comes from a slice of multi-grain bread or a cube of sugar; whether it comes from a fat-laden super-sized burger on a softball-sized white bun, or a salmon fillet. It. Still. Counts. The reason your bomb calorimeter is imperfect is because the results obtained from the contrasting samples, stated previously, do not yield the same results. Although the energy extracted from the contrasting samples is similar, one set of contrasting samples will cause you to die sooner and gain weight more easily; and the other set will allow you to live longer, better, and to lose weight faster and easier. I'll go out on a limb and guess that you know which are which. But we all know this already, right? I'm saying the same thing everyone else is saying, right?

The truth is: Some calories kill, some don't. If you want to live long and live well, you need to understand this. You need to keep reading. The truth will set you free.

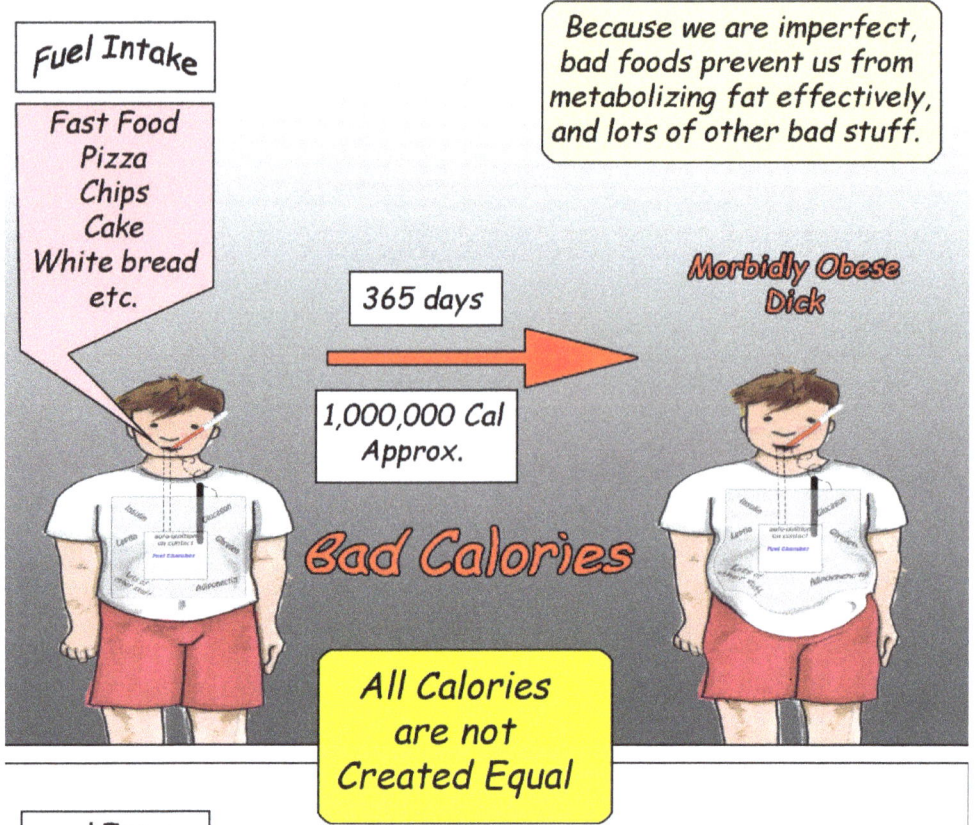

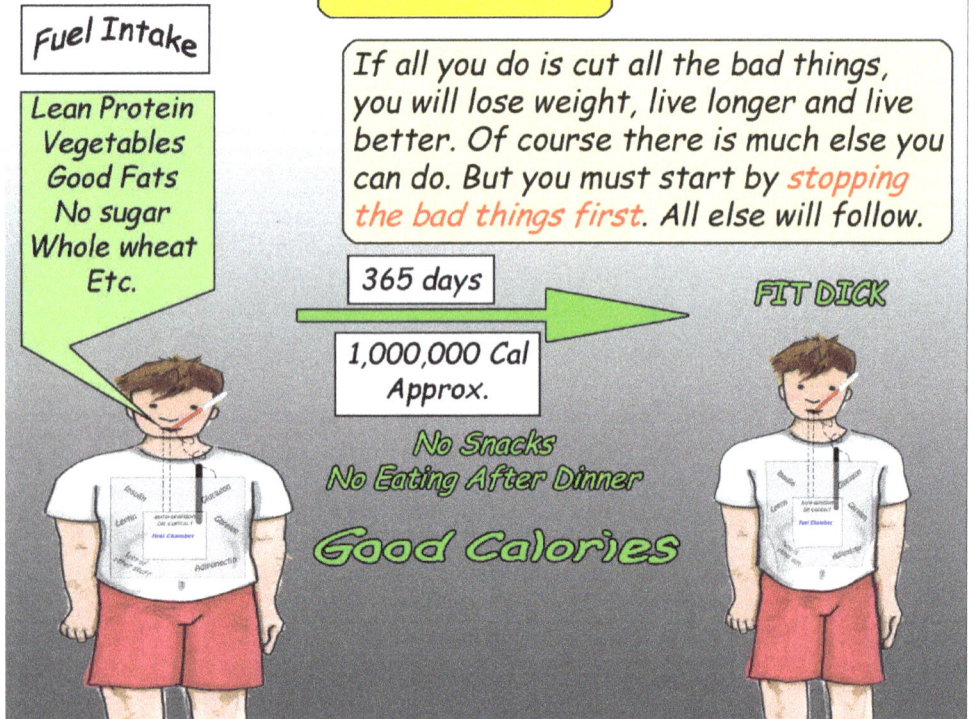

Phase II:

1. Understand the truth of a calorie.
2. **Establish your daily caloric need for a weight-loss of 1-2lbs./week.**
3. Be Accountable. Be Honest.
4. Get started by controlling the calories IN.

How many calories are the right amount? Can I eat as much as I want if they're good calories?

No. You can't eat as much as you want, even if they're good calories. You can eat more good calories than you can bad calories and still lose weight; but the energy still counts. *It's the law.* It is very simple to know how many calories you need to maintain your current weight. It is very simple to know how many calories you need to maintain your desired weight. These numbers will obviously be different, either by a lot if you are morbidly obese, or by a little if you are only overweight.

The back of a napkin number is 10 calories per pound per day; therefore, a 200-pound person needs about 2000 calories per day to maintain that weight. A more specific number can be obtained by punching numbers into an online caloric need calculator that uses the more scientific Harris-Benedict equation, which calculates your Basal Metabolic Rate (BMR). You can get a much more specific number based on your gender, age, and activity level at the National Institute of Health, National Institute of Diabetes and Digestive and Kidney Diseases, https://www.niddk.nih.gov/bwp.

> A **ROUGH APPROXIMATATION** OF **BASAL** CALORIC NEED IS **10 CAL/LB**; BUT THIS WILL UNDER-ESTIMATE YOUR TRUE NEED.

It is also the case that the generally accepted value of 3500 calories per pound of fat is very simplistic and of questionable utility in the imperfect bomb calorimeter; however, we're going to go with it, because it's easy and it works for the purposes of illustration, and more importantly, it will work with the strategies I am proposing.

> USE AN ON-LINE CALCULATOR FOR A MORE SPECIFIC MEASUREMENT OF YOUR DAILY CALORIC NEED. LINK AT FATTHIEF.COM.

Example: Consider an imperfect bomb calorimeter that is 5'7" and weighs 290 lbs. Those values yield a BMI of 45, which is extremely obese.

Using our *back of the napkin* numbers, because it's easier, to maintain that weight requires a daily intake of 2900 Calories. To get to a BMI of 25, which is one value into the *overweight category*, would require a weight-loss of 130 lbs. in order to get to 160. At 160 lbs. the daily requirement to maintain that weight would be 1600 Calories. Remember, this is strictly energy consideration, without accounting for the quality of the macronutrients.

If that is a new word for you, *macronutrients*, all I mean by that is that there are three broad classes of the foods (nutrients) we eat, and they are fats, carbohydrates (sugar), and protein.

The Macronutrients
Carbohydrate = 4 (4.1 actual) Calories/gram
Protein = 4 (4.35 actual) Calories/gram
Fat = 9 (9.3 actual) Calories/gram

You need to know that the daily caloric calculation above is based upon your basal metabolic needs. It does not account for the energy expended in exercise or the labor of work or walking 10,000 steps. It is primarily a calculation for a sedentary lifestyle. If you go from bed to breakfast to car to elevator to office chair, and then reverse order to dinner to bed; or if your primary pastime is binge watching Game of Thrones, from sun up to sun down; then your estimated daily caloric need is not too far off from this baseline calculation.

> The Macronutrients are ENERGY. They are FUEL for the body.
>
> If the fuel is not used. It must be stored. It's not going to evaporate.

That's great. So how much should I eat to lose weight?

Continuing with the example above (substitute your own numbers), you want to get from a BMI of 45 to a BMI of 25, which means a weight-loss of 130 pounds. One might think, that's easy, I'll just start eating the daily requirement for my goal weight of 160 pounds, which would be 1600 Cal/day. Unfortunately, it's not that easy. For one thing, you're talking about eating half of what you normally do and that may require more willpower than you presently have, and we will cross that bridge. Believe me. Besides that, it may not work as well as you think it would.

> REDUCE INTAKE 500 TO 1000 CALORIES/DAY TO ACHIEVE THE 1-2 LBS./WEEK TARGET.

> 3500 **CALORIES** IS ROUGHLY EQUIVELANT TO **1 LB. OF FAT;**
>
> SO, **500 CAL/D X 7D = 3500 CAL/WK**

Remember what I said about us being imperfect bomb calorimeters? We have all sorts of tricky things having to do with hormones and chemical mediators and metabolism. What do you think that little gland called the hypothalamus, in the middle bottom of your brain, is going to tell your body if you suddenly start eating half of what you used to, day after day? It's going to tell your body that you're absolutely starving, and your metabolism is going to slow down, which means that your imperfect bomb calorimeter is going to burn energy slower than it did before, and you will lose less weight than you think you should, given the assumption of 1 lb. = 3500 Cal.

You must do things in certain ways, and these will all be revealed shortly, and they will be, if not easy, at least *easier*; but, for now, in Phase II, set a relaxed goal of losing 1-2 pounds per week.

At 3500 Cal/pound of fat, this amounts to decreasing your calories by 500-1000 Calories/day. This would eventually bring you within spitting distance of your goal weight relative to where you started from, but there is still much more that you can do.

Phase II:

1. Understand the truth of a calorie.
2. Establish your daily caloric need for a weight-loss of 1-2lbs./week.
3. **Be Accountable. Be Honest.**
4. **Get started by controlling the calories IN.**

That sounds so EASY, but it's not. You must be accountable, and you must be honest.

You now know exactly what a calorie is and that you are imperfect in how you handle the calories that are only energy, albeit life-sustaining energy; however, you have to know exactly how many calories are in the food energy you are eating, if you don't already. As I initially described in the spectrum of diets, counting calories is less important with the extremes of low-fat/plant-based and low-carb/ketogenic diets, but they still do matter. If you have never counted calories and couldn't, off the top of your head, say how many calories are in a quarter cup of almonds, and how big that quarter cup is in the palm of your hand (hint: it's not as much as you think it is); then you should count calories and weigh your portion sizes with a food scale for two weeks. That is all I ask. It will be instructive and serve as a reference point. I haven't routinely counted calories for years, but I still add things up at times when they seem too good to be true, and they always are. It is always more than you think, unless it doesn't taste great, then it's probably OK.

Counting calories and weighing your food for accurate portion sizes is being accountable to yourself. You need to teach yourself these things. Only you can do it. When you weigh out 2 ounces of whole wheat pasta, which is considered one serving, you will see what I mean. You will learn that a smallish chicken breast weighs about 4 ounces and has about 184 calories. This would be a broiled, baked, sautéed skinless chicken breast.

How many calories do you think are in one piece of an eight-piece bucket of a popular fast food establishment? An extra-crispy, breast on the bone, contains **530 Calories**.

START A FOOD JOURNAL

COUNTING CALORIES, KEEPING A FOOD JOURNAL, IS ONE OF THE BEST THINGS YOU CAN DO BECAUSE ONLY THEN WILL YOU LEARN WHAT A TRUE PORTION SIZE IS.

IT IS NOT FOREVER, ONLY AS LONG AS IT TAKES YOU TO LEARN WHAT IS RIGHT AND WHAT IS WRONG.

Did you ever eat just one piece of fried chicken from a bucket of the same...? I didn't think so. *Did you completely strip off the skin and all breading and then squish out some of the grease from the deep-fried exposed meat with a napkin before you ate it?* Mmm, hmmm; of course not: Why would you? People would stare; besides, that's the whole point of fried chicken in the first place, isn't it? That crispy deep-fried-ness.

Keeping track of calories is much easier than it used to be if you have a smart phone because all you need is an app *(MyFitnessPal, My Plate)*, and there are several, free, that work well. In addition to that, every food you buy from the store, other than produce or meat, will have a label. You may have to weigh a portion size or use a measuring cup for pasta or rice, but most likely you won't be eating much of that anyway. The objective is to be accountable to yourself, to be honest with yourself, and in doing that you will learn the caloric content and the visual representation of appropriate portion sizes of the foods you eat.

Now. It is time for you to take control.

You know what to do to get started, and you should do it in this order, for several reasons.

REASONS TO DO IT IN THIS ORDER

1. IT'S IMPORTANT TO START AT THE BEGINNING WITH THE OBVIOUS EASY THINGS FIRST.
2. IT WILL WORK FOR A MAJORITY OF PEOPLE.
3. IT'S LESS OF A CHANGE FROM WHAT YOU ARE PROBABLY ALREADY DOING.
4. YOU DO WANT TO LOSE WEIGHT GRADUALLY OVER TIME TO ALLOW YOUR SKIN ELASTICITY TO COMPENSATE FOR YOUR SHRINKING VOLUME AND YOU'RE LESS LIKELY TO NEED A PANNICULECTOMY (CUTTING OFF LOOSE BELLY SKIN, WHICH IS CALLED A *PANNUS*). YOU DON'T WANT A *PANNUS PROBLEM*, STILL, IT'S NOTHING AN OPERATION WON'T FIX.
5. IT'S SAFE.

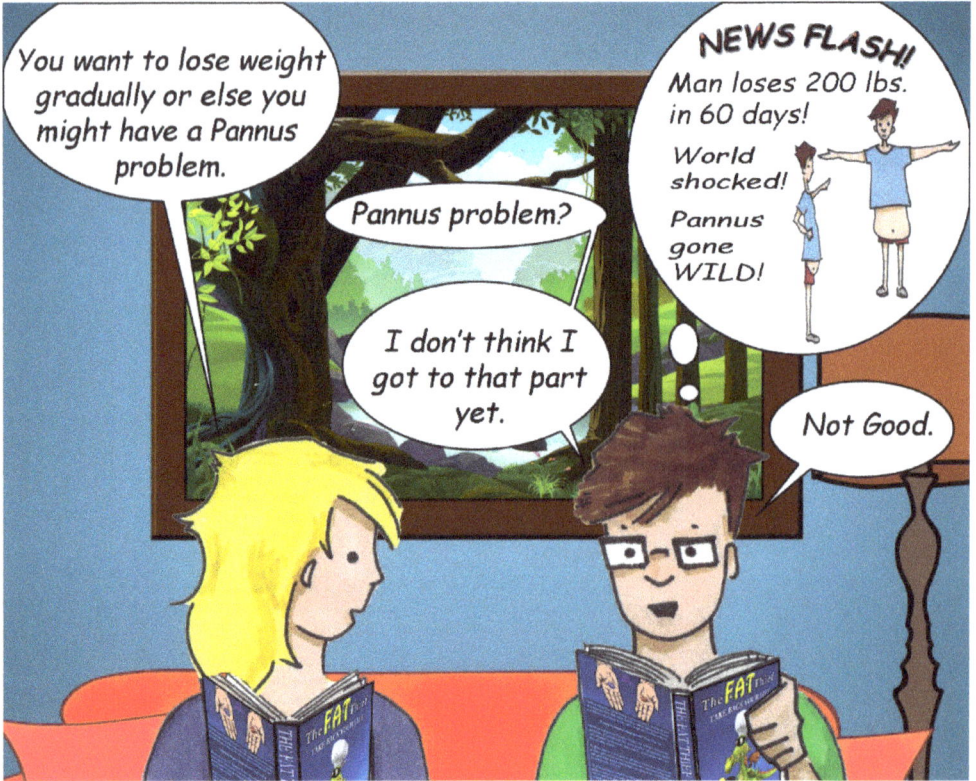

ANY TIME YOU SIGNIFICANTLY CHANGE YOUR DIET, AND ARE TAKING PRESCRIPTION MEDICATIONS FOR DIABETES, HYPERTENSION, HEART OR LUNG DISEASE, OR OTHER CHRONIC ILLNESSES, **YOU MUST DISCUSS AND REVIEW YOUR INTENT AND OBJECTIVES WITH YOUR PRIMARY CARE PROVIDER** BECAUSE IF YOU FOLLOW THESE GUIDELINES, YOU WILL LOSE WEIGHT AND THE MEDICATIONS YOU ARE CURRENTLY TAKING MIGHT CAUSE YOU HARM BECAUSE YOU *MAY NOT NEED THEM ANY LONGER*, OR AT LEAST, AS MUCH.

In Summary

1. PICK A DIET PLAN: MY BIAS IS TOWARDS A LOW-CARB KETOGENIC, ANTI-INFLAMMATORY STRATEGY. IT IS MY FEELING THAT THESE DIETS ARE EASIER TO COMPLY WITH AS THEY ARE LESS RESTRICTIVE THAN THE PLANT-BASED, ANIMAL-PRODUCT-AVOIDANCE STRATEGY; BUT, YOU'RE THE BOSS. PICK WHATEVER YOU WANT.
2. PREPARE YOUR CASTLE: MAKE YOUR HOME A SAFE PLACE. IT IS YOUR FORTRESS OF SOLITUDE THAT SHOULD BE IMPERVIOUS TO THE DRAGON. HAVE A STRATEGY FOR HOW YOU'RE GOING TO EAT WHEN OUTSIDE THE WALL.
3. USE AN ONLINE BASAL CALORIC NEED CALCULATOR TO FIGURE OUT HOW MANY CALORIES YOU SHOULD CONSUME PER DAY TO LOSE 1-2 POUNDS PER WEEK: IF YOU ARE ON ONE OF THE DIETS TOWARDS EITHER EXTREME OF LOW-FAT, PLANT-BASED; OR, LOW-CARB KETOGENIC, COUNTING CALORIES IS LESS IMPORTANT, BUT I THINK IT IS STILL HELPFUL FOR A FEW WEEKS, UNTIL YOU HAVE AN APPRECIATION OF HOW MANY CALORIES ARE IN THE FOODS YOU EAT. <HTTPS://WWW.NIDDK.NIH.GOV/BWP>
4. BE HONEST. BE TRUE TO YOURSELF. CONTROL WHAT YOU EAT.

Welcome to the end of Phase II. What I have described above is the basic, caloric-controlled standard diet that is common among all those diets in the middle in which there are significant proportions of all three of the basic macronutrients (fats, protein, carbohydrates) in which counting calories is crucial. Unfortunately, this conventional, caloric-restricted, calorie-counting diet doesn't work for some because of a disrupted metabolism from previous efforts of caloric restriction, poor macronutrient selection, or any host of other reasons.

There remains the inalienable truth that we are imperfect bomb calorimeters, and as such, one type of calorie does not necessarily equal another even though they both contain the same amount of energy. Certain calories will exert unfavorable effects on your metabolism whereas others will not. Certain calories will exert unfavorable systemic effects by inducing an inflammatory-prone state leading to disease and death whereas others will not. You must know the difference.

It is this way because that is how we are made. We are built to live long and live lean; we are built to efficiently store massive amounts of energy for future famine: we are built to efficiently expend great amounts of energy over extended periods of time; what I mean by this is that we gain weight easy and we lose weight hard. Now, we're going to take it up a notch. This requires you to be more smarter ;^) so time to put a few more bricks into the WALL....

> A BASIC CALORIC RESTRICTED DIET DOES NOT WORK FOR EVERYONE.
>
> DIFFERENT STRATEGIES MAY BE REQUIRED.
>
> YOU NEED TO OUTSMART YOUR METABOLISM.

CHAPTER FIVE: Phase III: Insulin, Metabolism, and Death

Phase III:

1. Understand the truth of insulin.
2. Control your carbohydrates.
3. Introduce an extended overnight fast.
4. Introduce a super-extended overnight fast.
5. Understand the truth that Obesity kills.

In Phase I and Phase II, you learned the basic diet strategy that is built around a caloric-restricted diet of otherwise healthy foods. Naturally, there are a ton of other diets, and fad diets that I'm not going to mention. The sole focus will be on what works and why it works. After these initial phases of learning, you are like a yellow belt in Karate and now it's time for your green belt. Poor dragon.

The first part of Phase III, the truth about insulin, is probably the most difficult but also the most important part of this first arrow of truth with which you will render a mortal blow to the dragon. I want this to be so obvious and clear to you that to not respect the truth would be, in effect, a form of self-immolation in which you are knowingly causing harm to yourself, as is the case with smoking, excessive drinking and any other harmful habits or addictions.

I am going to use deductive logic, like solving a Euclidian geometry problem, and it's okay if you don't remember that. In deductive reasoning, one draws a conclusion from known truths or givens; therefore, we will start with the truths. These will be grossly simplified; however, that does not mean that they are not true. *They are most definitely true.* Although these truths or givens are not universal laws like the previously mentioned first law of thermodynamics that deals with the conservation of energy, or the speed of light in a vacuum; they are as valid and could be considered biological truths or biological laws. We must learn to respect the laws for they are part of the first arrow; the arrow of truth.

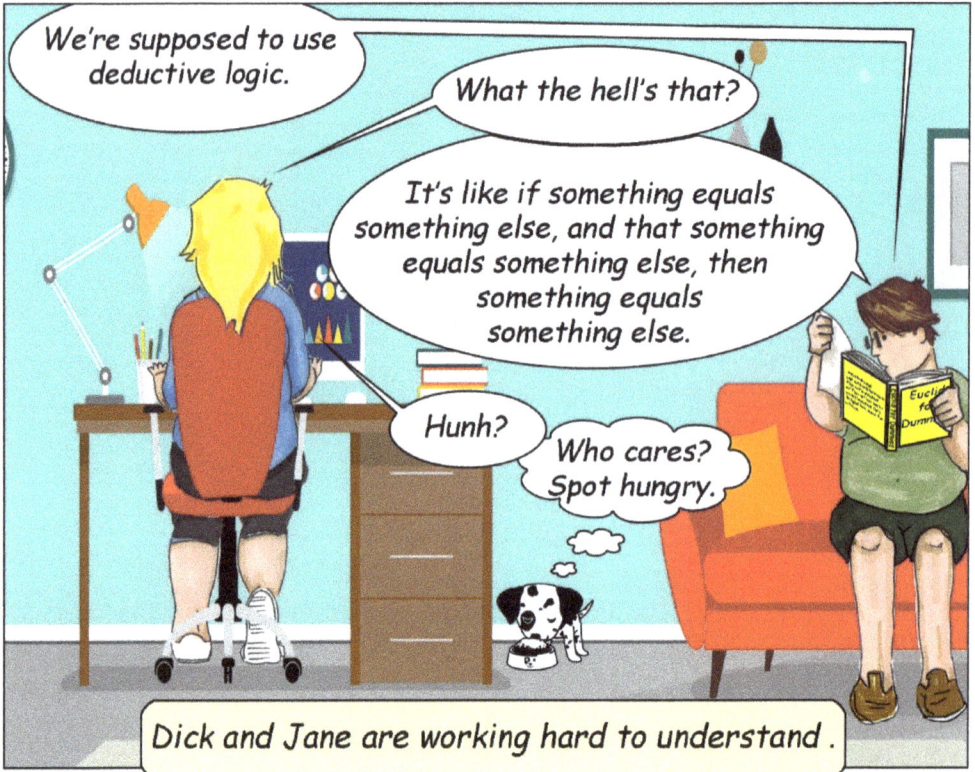

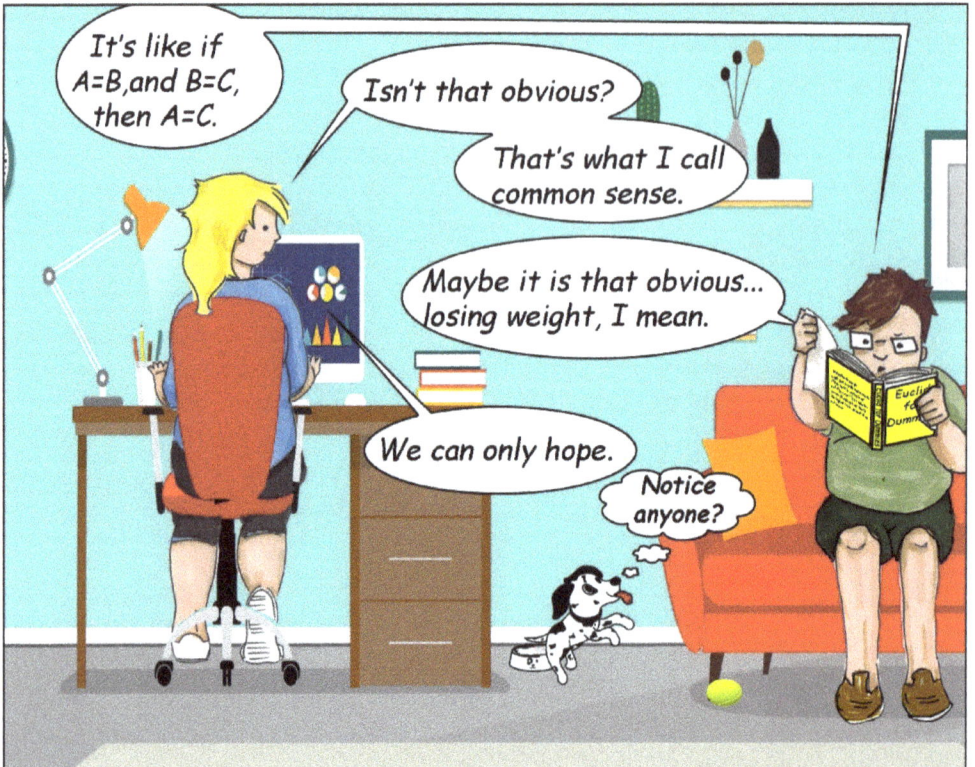

Phase III:

1. Understand the truth of insulin.
2. Control your carbohydrates.
3. Introduce an extended overnight fast.
4. Introduce a super-extended overnight fast.
5. Understand the truth that Obesity kills.

Metabolism refers to the chemical processes that occur in a living organism to maintain life. You can think of it as "burning." You can metabolize/burn carbohydrate or fat or protein for energy needs of the body.

We will now be learning of the **_Seven Biological Truths_** that impact your metabolism and how your body uses and stores energy. These truths are the givens with which we will construct our deductive arguments. All this information is generally accepted basic science information (unless otherwise referenced), as might be found in a general textbook of medical physiology, such as the one I learned from, Guyton's (1). As I have said, and as I will continue to say, this manual is a manual of absolutes. There is much more nuance and complexity involved in all these processes, but I am painting a picture for you in bold colors and with broad strokes. The real picture is intricately much more beautiful.

BIOLOGICAL TRUTH #1
INSULIN TURNS OFF FAT METABOLISM AND STORES ENERGY (FOOD) AS FAT OR GLYCOGEN.

Insulin is a hormone secreted by the beta cells of the pancreas: It builds tissue up (anabolic). It does not break tissue down (catabolic). It turns all excess ingested macronutrients into stored energy (**fat/glycogen**). In other words: **Insulin makes fat.**

Insulin suppresses fat metabolism: Since it is anabolic and builds up and does not tear down, when insulin is present in the blood, it is not possible to metabolize/burn fat to a significant degree. It does the opposite. It builds up fat.

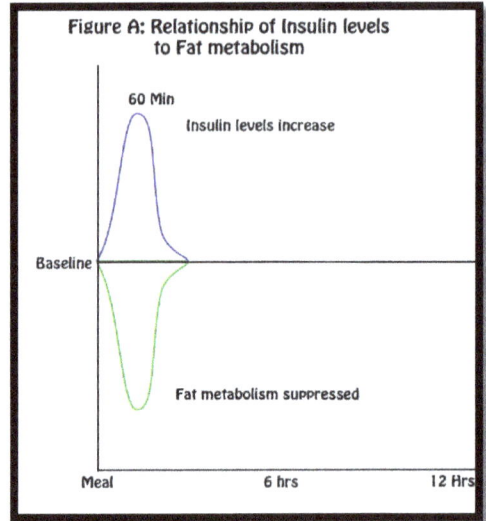

Figure A: Relationship of Insulin levels to Fat metabolism

60 Min

Insulin levels increase

Baseline

Fat metabolism suppressed

Meal   6 hrs   12 Hrs

This truth is listed first because it is primary. It is the key to understanding the reason why one calorie does not necessarily equal another when your goal is to lose weight, or in other words *metabolize fat*. Some calories cause the release of insulin and when insulin is present in the blood stream, fat is not metabolized or burned, it is added to, fat is stored, fat is built up, that is what insulin does, it builds up, it does not tear down.

BIOLOGICAL TRUTH #2
CARBOHYDRATE/SUGAR IS THE PRIMARY MACRONUTRIENT THAT CAUSES THE RELEASE OF INSULIN.

Carbohydrate is the primary macronutrient that causes the release of insulin: Sugar and refined carbohydrates (high-glycemic) cause the quickest and the most release of insulin into the blood stream. The carbohydrate of a peach or sweet potato (lower-glycemic) also causes a release of insulin, but slower and not as much.

Glucose is **Sugar** is **Carbohydrate**. They are interchangeable. After a meal of **Carbohydrate**, the **Insulin** levels peak at 30-60 minutes and drops about eighty percent over the next three hours.

BIOLOGICAL TRUTH #3
PROTEIN ALSO CAUSES THE RELEASE OF INSULIN, NOT AS MUCH AS CARBOHYDRATES, BUT IT STILL DOES.

Protein is also a macronutrient that causes the release of insulin: It does not cause as much insulin to be released, or as quickly as does carbohydrates; but it still does. Eating a high-protein diet does not accomplish weight-loss by itself--all the excess protein, not used by the body for metabolic needs, is converted into glucose for storage (fat).

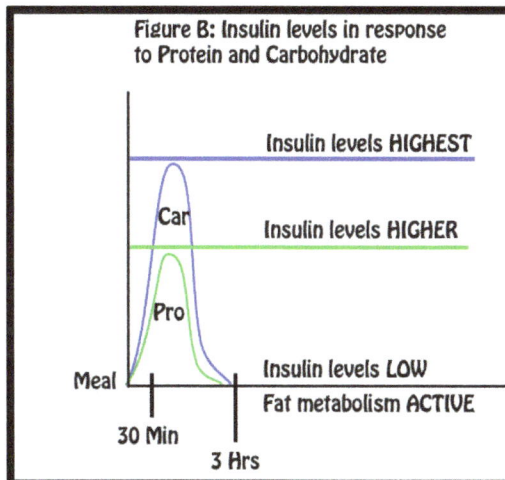

Figure B: Insulin levels in response to Protein and Carbohydrate

Insulin levels HIGHEST

Car

Insulin levels HIGHER

Pro

Insulin levels LOW

Fat metabolism ACTIVE

Meal

30 Min

3 Hrs

> ### BIOLOGICAL TRUTH #4
>
> FAT IS STORED ENERGY. IT DOES NOT CAUSE A SIGNIFICANT RELEASE OF INSULIN IF INGESTED.

Fat, when ingested, does not cause a significant release of insulin; but how often do you eat fat alone? Probably not very often. It is likely that you eat either carbohydrate or protein with the fat, and that means you will be releasing insulin into the blood; furthermore, there is an enhanced response to the release of insulin with the ingestion of both carbohydrate *and* fat. (2) What this means is that eating fat with carbohydrates is worse than eating carbohydrates alone from the standpoint of the amount of insulin released and the realization of Biological Truth #1:--insulin turns fat metabolism off--instead, the extra insulin released makes even more fat from the ingested carbohydrate and fat.

> ### BIOLOGICAL TRUTH #5
>
> GLYCOGEN IS STORED ENERGY. IT IS THE STORAGE FORM OF CARBOHYDRATE/GLUCOSE.

Glycogen is the storage form of carbohydrate: Most of the body's glycogen stores are in the liver and muscle. **Glycogen** is *stored* energy, as is fat. The structure of **Glycogen** is that of a multibranched chain made of **glucose** molecules all linked together.

> ### BIOLOGICAL TRUTH #6
>
> INSULIN TURNS NEARLY ALL INGESTED FOOD NOT USED FOR METABOLIC NEEDS INTO GLUCOSE, THEN INTO GLYCOGEN, THEN INTO FAT, *IN THAT ORDER.*

Insulin turns ingested macronutrients not used for ongoing metabolism into stored energy: It turns ingested **carbohydrates** into **glycogen**, then into fat, *in that order.* It turns ingested protein not used for bodily protein synthesis into **carbohydrate**, then into **glycogen**, then into fat, *in that order.* It turns ingested fat, not used for ongoing metabolism, into fat.

> ## BIOLOGICAL TRUTH #7
>
> ### YOUR BODY WILL ALWAYS BURN GLUCOSE FIRST, WHEN GIVEN THE CHOICE.

Your body will always burn/metabolize **Glucose** first when given the choice, then glycogen, and only then will it burn fat.

What happens when you eat more than you metabolize?

The short answer: You make fat.

The longer answer: **Ingested carbohydrates** cause the release of insulin from the pancreas. As an anabolic hormone, insulin's function is to build up, so it does this in a very specific order. First, it converts circulating glucose (very quickly) into glycogen; then, when all the glycogen stores in the liver and muscle are filled up, it will convert all the excess carbohydrates to fat. Since insulin suppresses fat metabolism, **it is literally impossible for you to significantly metabolize any of your fat stores when insulin (above baseline) is present in your bloodstream.**

Ingested protein also causes the release of insulin; not as much, however the circulating insulin does still suppress fat metabolism to some extent. Inside the intestinal tract, the protein is broken down into smaller molecules (peptides, amino acids) that are used for the daily protein needs for the maintenance and health of multiple organ systems. The excess protein molecules are then converted into glucose and then into glycogen, and then into fat when the glycogen stores are filled up, *in that order.*

> Every macronutrient you consume, all the energy that you eat, is absorbed by you, imperfect bomb calorimeter that you are. When your body is presented with energy in the form of fat, carbohydrate and protein, it will burn the carbohydrate first for current metabolic needs, then it will fill up your glycogen stores, then it will make fat.

As per *Biological Truth #4*, **Ingested fat** does not cause the release of insulin; however, typically you have also ingested carbohydrates and/or protein as well, so there will be some circulating insulin. The fat is broken down into smaller molecules (fatty acids) in the intestine and adsorbed into the blood. If there is circulating glucose, it is burned preferentially for current metabolic needs, and all the fatty acids are moved into fat storage because fat metabolism is suppressed. If there is no circulating glucose (no insulin), and if the glycogen stores are relatively depleted, then the fatty acids are utilized for current energy needs, then, any excess is moved into fat storage.

If you haven't noticed, *I know you have*, there runs through this a common thread. **If your glycogen stores are already filled up, then everything over and above your current needs will go directly to fat**; so, basically, most everything you eat will turn into fat *if your glycogen stores are filled up*, unless you happen to be running a marathon concurrently.

You're probably wondering: *How big are my glycogen stores?* About 500 grams, give or take, depending on your weight. Although the liver has the highest concentration of glycogen (6-10% weight), it is the muscle that contains most of the glycogen (1-2% weight). Since all the muscles in the body represent a larger mass than the liver, the muscle contains 80% of the body's glycogen stores. 500 grams is not a lot, about 2000 Calories; one day in the wilderness with nothing but a canteen of water; two to three hours of aerobic exercise, and it's gone.

For the sake of contrast, consider the amount of energy in your body's fat stores given that an acceptable body-fat percent is 25-32% of body weight. For a 150-pound woman with 30% body-fat that would be 45 pounds at 3500 Calories per pound, or, 157,500 Calories. That's a lot of energy. Here's a math problem for you. Add up how many calories you might eat on Thanksgiving Day. Assume that your glycogen stores are full. How many pounds of extra fat do you wake up with after a day of continuous eating (the old you) while watching the Macy's Day Parade, the National Dog Show, and then football, all from a horizontal position?

Your glycogen stores of about 2000 Calories are like your checking account, you keep enough in there to manage day-to-day. Your fat stores contain enormous amounts of energy, 50-200,000 Calories, or more; they are like your savings account, you only access them when your checking account is depleted.

Energy buckets and a math problem.

Before leaving the topic of energy metabolism, Thanksgiving and football, I want to see if I can make this all a little more real with an analogy. I want this to be crystal clear, like one of those full moons in October with an orange-cratered face suspended above the horizon like it's about to fall to earth at any moment. Crystal. Like that.

I'll call this my *energy bucket analogy* and will represent it graphically at the end, but before getting into it we need to establish a few givens:

GIVENS
1) AVERAGE FASTING BLOOD GLUCOSE = 70-99 MG/DL (MILLIGRAMS PER DECILITER, WHICH IS $1/10^{TH}$ OF A LITER).   2) VOLUME OF BLOOD IN A 70KG MALE = 5 LITERS.   3) BASAL METABOLIC RATE (BMR) FOR A 70KG PERSON = 1600 CAL./DAY.   4) 24 HRS/DAY = 1440 MINUTES/DAY; THEREFORE, BMR FOR A 70KG PERSON = 1.1 CAL./MINUTE.

The energy we consume and expend and store exists in four compartments, *or buckets*, within our body; the blood glucose bucket, the glycogen bucket, the fat bucket, and the protein bucket, in that order, from the top down, and energy flows between the buckets, like water down a fall.

The protein bucket doesn't count so much as a form of energy storage as it is primarily involved in the functions of the various organ systems, however, it is accessed during the end-stages of starvation for energy needs, until the bodily functions become so impaired that the organism dies, as tragically demonstrated by the death of the well-known American singer, Karen Carpenter in 1983.

The first bucket, blood glucose, is really no bucket at all as it is so small, more a thimble really. It is closely connected to the glycogen bucket such that there is a free flow of glucose molecules back and forth, which keeps the blood glucose in a tight range of roughly 20-30 points on either side of 100 mg/dL.

MATH PROBLEM for Amt. of Glucose in Blood
80 MG GLU/DL X1GM/1000MG X 10DL/1L=0.8 GM GLU/L   0.8 GM GLU/L X 5 L BLOOD = **4 GM GLU** IN BLOOD STREAM

You need to understand how small this bucket is. From the above givens, you can derive the size of the bucket with a blood sugar of 80 (a normal fasting value) an easy math problem.

Any idea how much **four grams** *of sugar is?* Not a lot. A small sugar cube contains five grams. One teaspoon of sugar equals 4.2 grams. Now, consider that all ingested carbohydrate and some fraction of the protein enter via the blood glucose bucket. *The illustration of the little bucket to the right is not to scale. It is significantly smaller relative to the other illustrated buckets.*

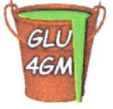

This means that the little bucket fills up very quickly when swamped with anything from a 100-calorie snack to a 2000 calorie dinner, or more. It then overflows into the next bucket (glycogen), and then into the next (fat).

The glycogen bucket is much larger. The glycogen stores in the liver (100gm) and the muscle (400gm) total 500gm, which equals 2000 calories of energy (4 cal./gm x 500gm). All the energy pouring into the blood stream from a meal or a snack must go somewhere. It cannot stay in the blood and it is the insulin that facilitates the movement of energy out of the blood and into the other buckets. The significance of the first bucket being so small is that pretty much all the energy consumed is moved, nearly immediately (1-3hrs), into the lower buckets. As soon as the glycogen bucket is filled, all energy flows into the next lower bucket, the fat bucket.

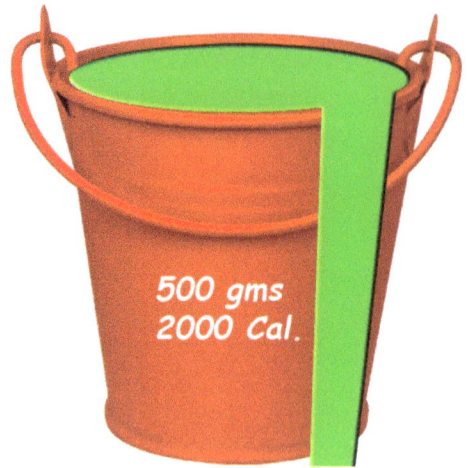

Because the basal metabolic rate (BMR) is a measly 1 Cal/minute, there is no significant burning of the energy being consumed for current metabolic needs as those needs are so minimal when compared to the comparatively vast quantities of hundreds of calories being consumed in the span of minutes.

A BMR of 1600 C/day equals only 1.1 Calories/minute.

This means that essentially all energy consumed during a meal is moved into storage, Glycogen first (if not already full), then Fat.

The fat bucket is by far the largest bucket, and there is *no limit to its potential size.* It is the endpoint for all excess energy that is consumed and not expended. All excess carbohydrates are easily converted to fat. All excess protein is easily converted to carbohydrate and then into fat, if not into glycogen first. All ingested fat is outside of the blood glucose bucket and is separately broken down and stored as fat in the liver (fatty liver) and, of course, in the body's places of fat accumulation.

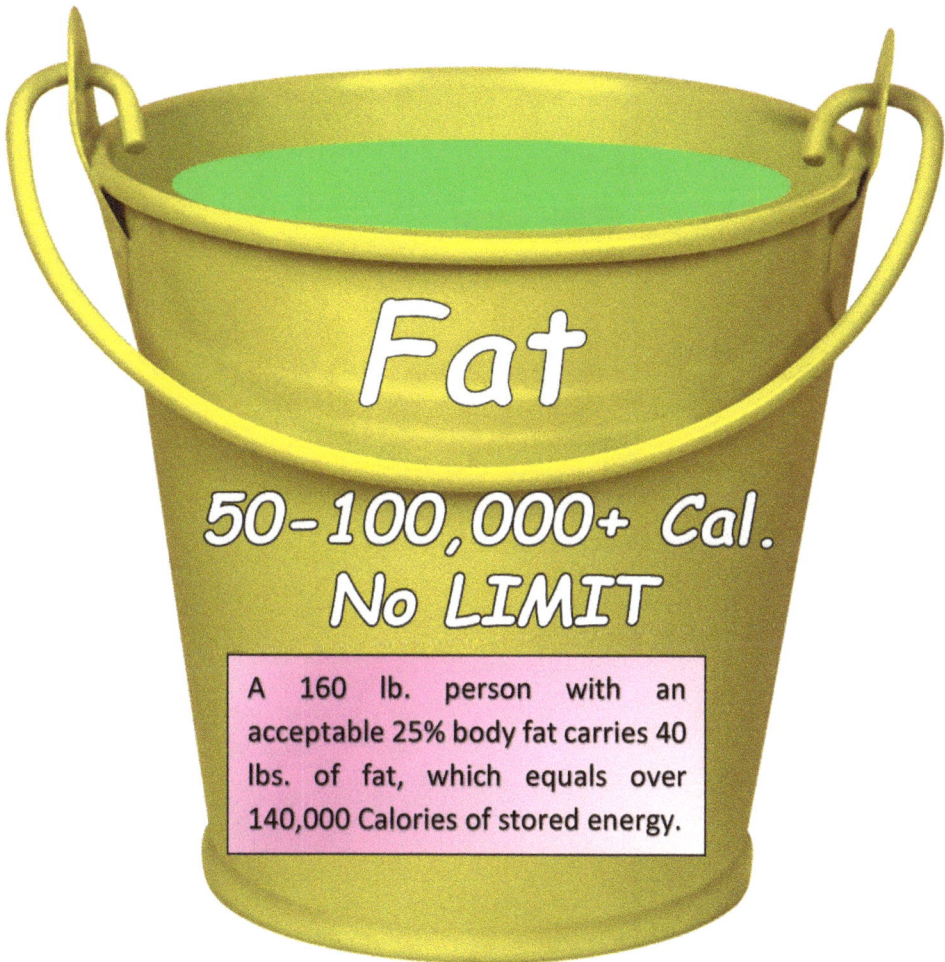

From the consumption standpoint and energy storage, the protein bucket does not apply so much as it is almost a separate bucket, but the other three buckets are closely connected and energy flows between them like water, filling them from the top down; the blood glucose bucket first, then the glycogen bucket, then the fat. **The fat bucket never fills up, it just gets larger, and larger, and larger.**

Please study the following diagram. Take your time. This needs to be clear.

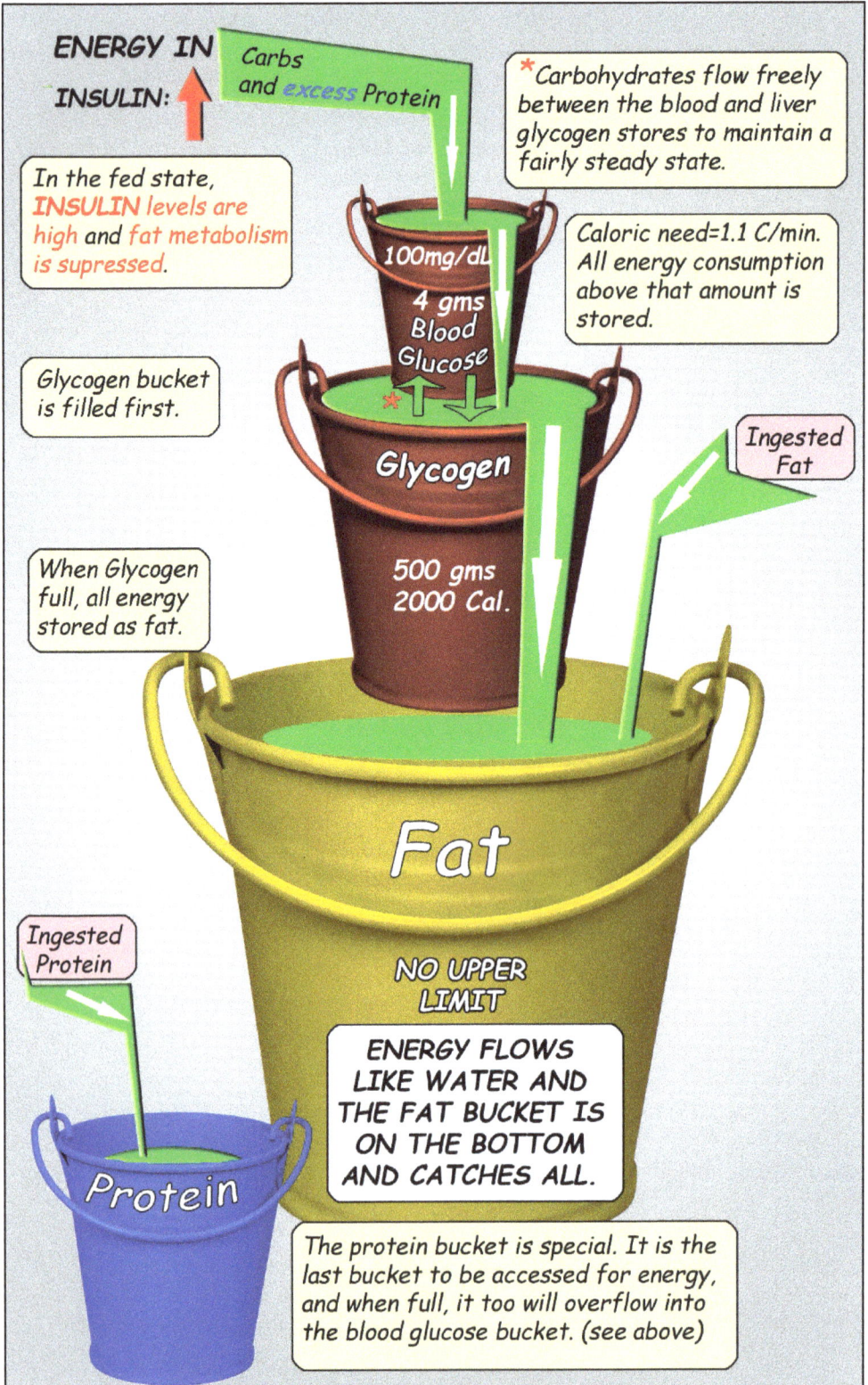

ENERGY IN

INSULIN:

Carbs and *excess* Protein

*Carbohydrates flow freely between the blood and liver glycogen stores to maintain a fairly steady state.

In the fed state, **INSULIN** levels are high and fat metabolism is supressed.

100mg/dL

4 gms Blood Glucose

Caloric need=1.1 C/min. All energy consumption above that amount is stored.

Glycogen bucket is filled first.

Glycogen

Ingested Fat

When Glycogen full, all energy stored as fat.

500 gms 2000 Cal.

Fat

Ingested Protein

NO UPPER LIMIT

ENERGY FLOWS LIKE WATER AND THE FAT BUCKET IS ON THE BOTTOM AND CATCHES ALL.

Protein

The protein bucket is special. It is the last bucket to be accessed for energy, and when full, it too will overflow into the blood glucose bucket. (see above)

Let us now look at the converse, when energy leaves the buckets.

Energy leaves the buckets in a similar fashion, from the top down. Glucose freely flows from the glycogen bucket into the much smaller blood glucose bucket as the glucose is *spent* at the cellular level. Remember that the glycogen is a multi-branching chain of glucose and the glucose molecules are chopped off the free ends of millions of trillions of branches of glycogen simultaneously and released into the blood. This is especially so during periods of activity, such as exercise, in which the glycogen stores in the liver and muscle are expended first, before the fat stores are accessed.

> At rest, the FAT bucket will be accessed directly for basal metabolic needs **UNLESS** there is circulating insulin from a meal or snack, which means fat metabolism will be suppressed.

At rest, the glycogen *and* fat stores are accessed for basal metabolic needs, so the energy requirements of the body at rest *are shared* between the glycogen bucket and the fat bucket. At night, during the fasting state, the glycogen bucket may be at least partially replenished by the metabolism of fat into glucose through the process of gluconeogenesis, and then into glycogen, so energy can not only flow directly from the fat bucket to the body, but also from the fat bucket to the glycogen bucket, if at rest.

Again, please study the following diagram. The important point, and I know I'm being repetitive, is that *as long as you keep the glycogen bucket full by eating frequently, especially by eating high-glycemic carbs (sugar equivalents), you will have persistently elevated insulin levels which will suppress fat metabolism and the fat bucket is rarely touched for energy.* It stays the same or it gets bigger if you eat more than you metabolize.

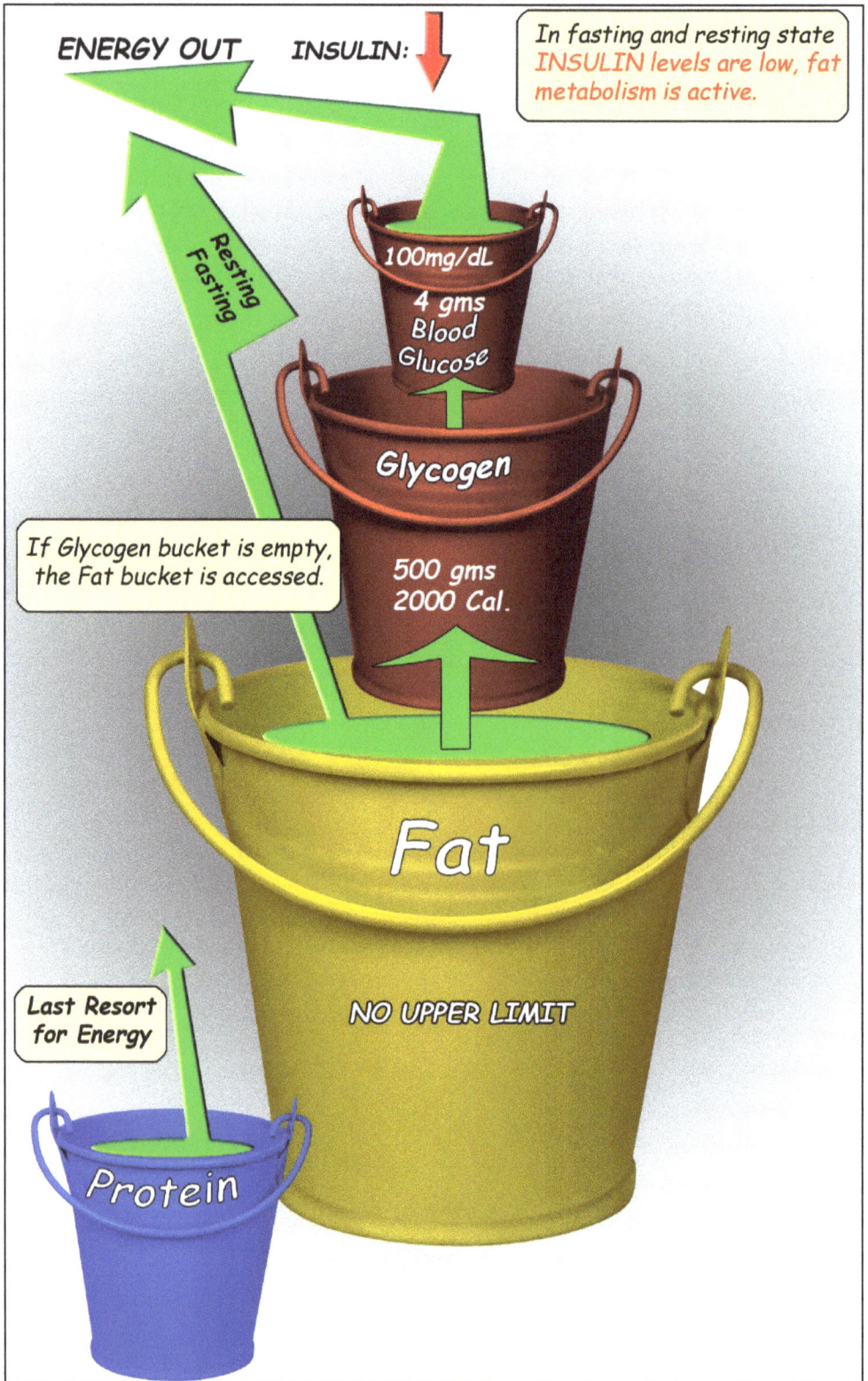

ENERGY OUT   INSULIN:

In fasting and resting state INSULIN levels are low, fat metabolism is active.

Resting
Fasting

100mg/dL
4 gms
Blood
Glucose

Glycogen

If Glycogen bucket is empty, the Fat bucket is accessed.

500 gms
2000 Cal.

Fat

NO UPPER LIMIT

Last Resort
for Energy

Protein

The reason I belabor this point is to illustrate the factual reality of how our bodies handle energy and with an eye on the prize of spending down the fat bucket. From all of the above, it should be patently obvious that if you keep your glycogen bucket full all of the time by frequent meals and snacks, especially those higher in carbohydrates, you will never access the fat bucket, unless you are in a significant caloric deficit. If that is the case and it is prolonged more than a few days, your body will interpret that as starvation, and it will lower your metabolic rate. You will conserve more energy and increase the tendency to store more fat, and weight-loss becomes that much more difficult.

I don't want to leave you with the impression that the fat bucket is bad. Nay, it is good. It is the fat bucket that has kept us alive through the millennium. We are not made to eat six, or even three times a day. We were built to starve intermittently. We were created to survive.

Recall the study I referenced in the 4th Biological Truth regarding fat metabolism. It showed that the release of insulin from carbohydrate ingestion was enhanced by also ingesting fat at the same time. You need to understand that our bodies are all about energy and survival, and from the evolutionary standpoint, fat is beautiful. Fat means survival, so when a caveman or cavewoman ate fat and carbohydrates, the insulin surge was greater so that the organism could store up even more of all that beautiful fat. That's how your body thinks. *Fat is beautiful.* Fat is the best storage form of energy, and, when burning energy stores, it saves the best bucket for last.

In way of illustration, let us consider Jesus, a Jewish male. From paintings, sculptures and crucifixes, and Jim Caviezel in *The Passion*, I'd guess maybe 170 pounds and 12% body fat at the time of his meeting with John the Baptist at the river Jordan. Do the math and you get about 70,000 calories, which runs to 1700 calories for each day of 40 in the wilderness. Plenty.

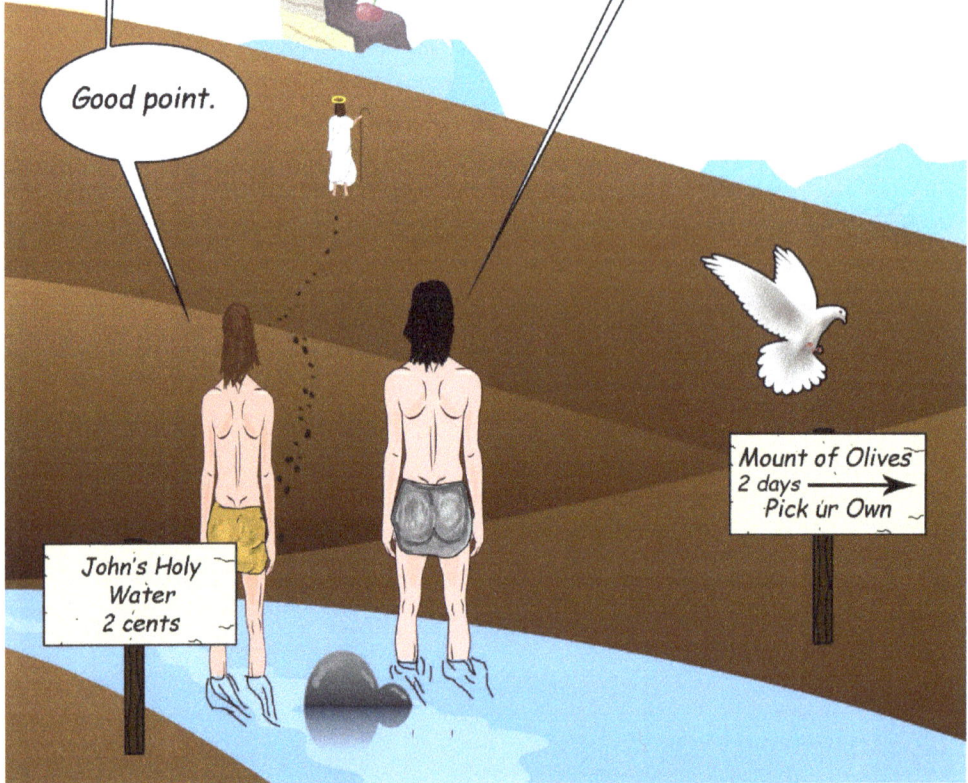

On becoming a more perfect bomb calorimeter.

I would suggest that you can become a more perfect bomb calorimeter relative to the burning of fat by utilizing the above truths. **It is time to draw some conclusions** from your newfound knowledge. It is time for you to be smarter than your metabolism. It is time to be like a ninja, even if a newly minted yellow belt, and begin sneaking up on the dragon.

Conclusion #1
SUGAR AND REFINED CARBOHYDRATES (WHITE FLOUR, WHITE RICE, PASTA, PASTRIES, ETC.) ARE FOOD OF THE DEVIL AND ARE TO BE AVOIDED.

Perhaps I have over-exaggerated in my exuberance; however, raw sugar and the highly refined carbohydrates of white bread, white pasta, white potatoes--let's just say everything that's white and soft and tastes great is bad. If it's white and crunchy and you have to chew it significantly before you swallow it, and it doesn't cause your eyes to roll back in an orgasmic gastronomical spasm of pleasure, it's probably okay. Radishes come to mind. And cauliflower.

But, what's Biological Truth #2 say? Carbohydrates cause the release of insulin. And what does insulin do? Insulin suppresses fat metabolism. You eat carbohydrates, you release insulin, you stop metabolizing fat. Instead, you make a little glycogen, then a lot of fat, unless you are burning the carbohydrates concurrently, like running a marathon.

Conclusion #2

INSULIN MAKES YOU FAT.

Please remember. My diet manual is an emphatic simplification, but I think it's effective when making these crucial points. To be clear, we are dependent on insulin. We need it. It was given to us by God, or evolution, or some combination of both, along with lots of other stuff; but we don't want *too much* insulin for *too long*.

Type 1 diabetics, Juvenile Diabetes, do not make enough insulin because the cells in the pancreas that make the insulin are destroyed. *Type 1 diabetics have low insulin levels* (don't make enough) and *are skinny*. In type 1 diabetics, the blood sugars are high because there isn't enough insulin to move it into glycogen and fat.

In type 2 diabetes the tissues are resistant to insulin and the normal amount that the pancreas makes is not enough and the pancreas can't keep up. The blood sugar is high because the body's tissues are resistant to the insulin, and *the insulin levels are higher* because the tissues need more insulin to bring down the blood sugars. Often, type 2 diabetics require extra insulin injected daily or oral medications that increase the body's sensitivity to insulin. *Type 2 diabetics are generally overweight or obese.*

The disease of diabetes illustrates the link between insulin and the metabolism of fat. Type 1 diabetics have low insulin levels and are thin; type 2 diabetics have high insulin levels and are overweight, in general.

Insulin makes you fat because when present, it keeps you from burning fat for energy, and it turns everything you eat, not being used directly for cellular metabolic needs, into fat. Insulin is both the answer and the problem, and by that, I mean to say *if you can recognize that insulin is the problem*, and then control it, you solve it.

In **Type 2 Diabetes** more insulin is needed because the tissues are resistant to it. This resistance is closely associated with obesity.

A type 2 diabetic can decrease their need for insulin by lowering their carbohydrate intake. In the process, they will lose weight and decrease the need for insulin, which is why weight-loss in diabetics requires close medical supervision.

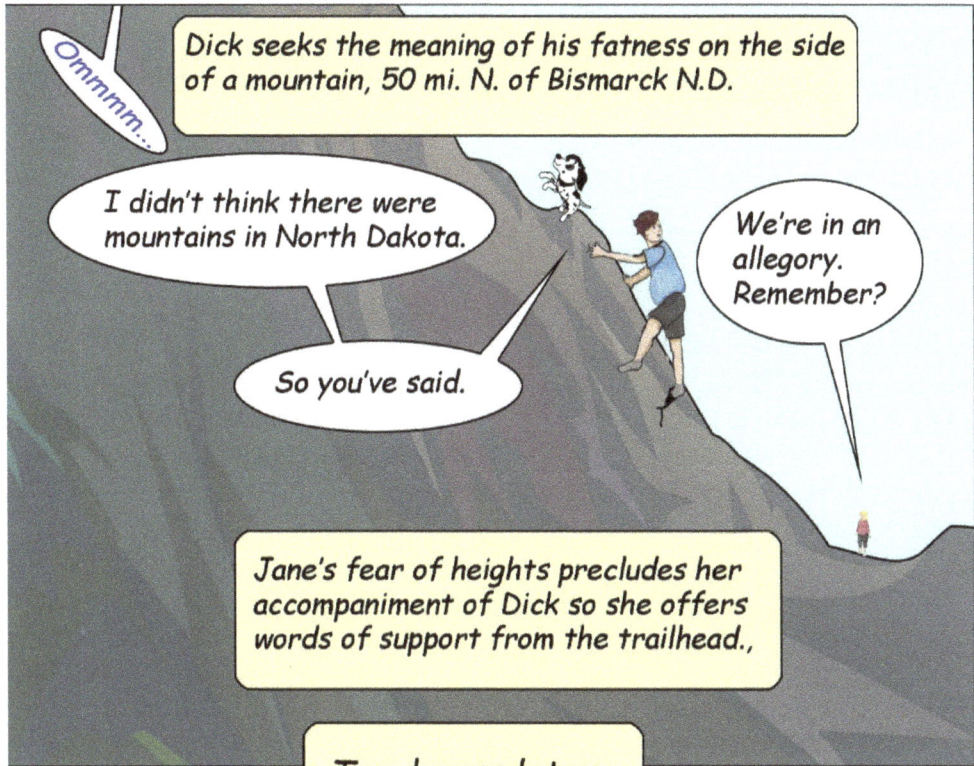

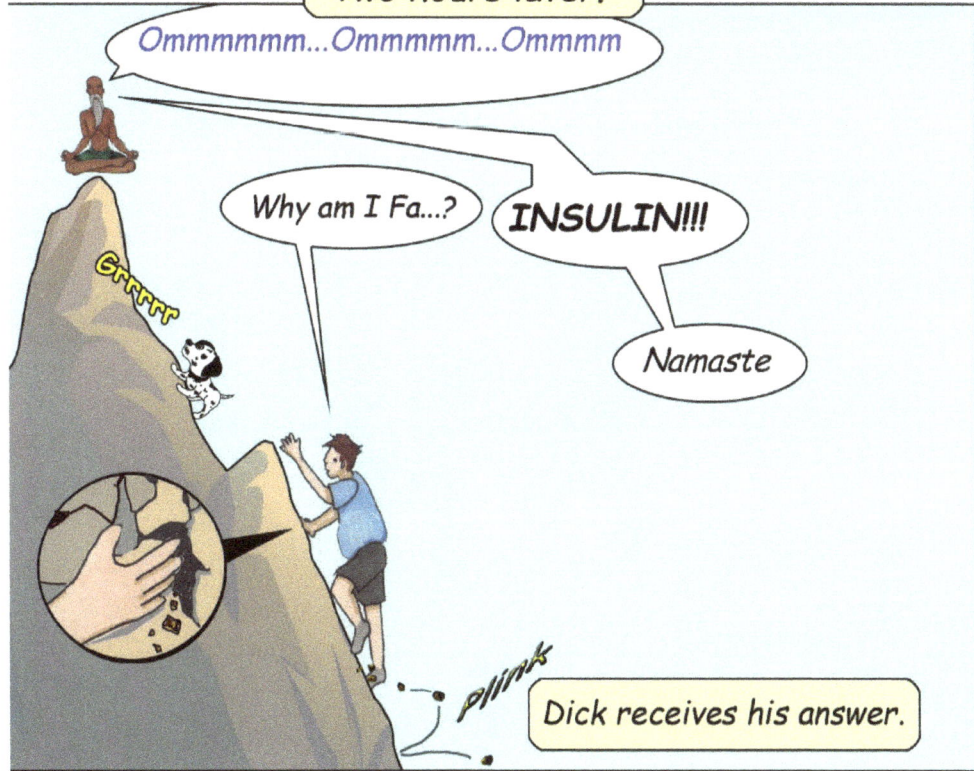

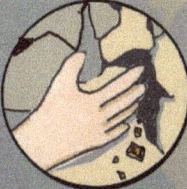

Conclusion #3

YOUR BODY WILL ALWAYS CHOOSE CARBOHYDRATE OVER FAT AS A FUEL SOURCE IF IT CAN.

This is not so much a conclusion as it is a fact, but it is such an important truth that it bears repetition. If you have carbohydrate meals for breakfast, lunch and dinner, and then some snacks in between, on breaks, or whatever, you will rarely burn fat during waking hours because of the steady state of elevated insulin levels in the blood stream. Your body has a very specific preference for energy needs. It will utilize circulating glucose first, then it will spend down the glucose in the glycogen stores in the liver and muscle; only then will it begin to burn fat to a significant extent.

With frequent eating, the blood levels of insulin never fall back to baseline during waking hours, with the result being a continuous suppression of fat metabolism until three hours after eating the last meal or snack of the day. The diagram below is a typical pattern of eating, let's call it the *Typical American Diet*, (**TAD**), in which one eats three meals a day, snacks and something before bed.

The effect of frequent eating on fat metabolism: Bad

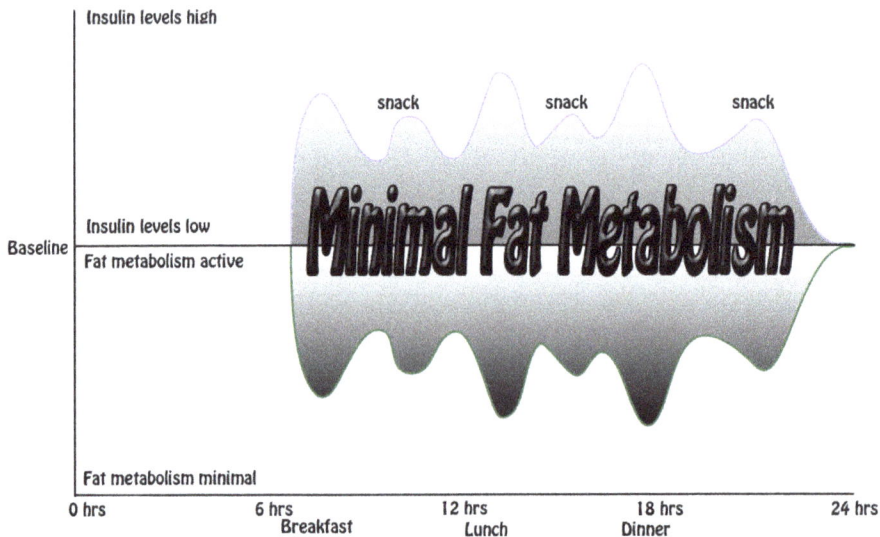

Conclusion #4

NIGHTTIME IS GOOD BECAUSE INSULIN LEVELS ARE LOW.

The body's natural tendency is to burn fat for metabolic needs at rest. If you are exercising at an exertional level beyond mild to moderate, your body will burn down its glycogen stores first and then shift to fat, but when you run out of glycogen your performance will suffer dramatically, which is why endurance athletes will hydrate with carbohydrate rich fluids and ingest carbohydrates during the course of a competition.

The natural tendency to burn fat at rest will be defeated by carbohydrate-rich meals and especially by consuming sugar (soda), sweets and highly refined carbohydrates. For an individual who eats carbohydrate meals and snacks or drinks carbohydrate rich liquids throughout the day, the only time they will metabolize fat to any significant extent is overnight, unless, of course, that individual keeps a box of Hostess Twinkies or equivalent on the nightstand. In that case they will never metabolize fat. Now, if that individual does not eat an excess of calories, then it may not be a problem for their weight; however, it is unhealthy and they likely will suffer the associated obesity-related diseases of the *skinny-fat*, skinny on the outside, fat on the inside, but that is another issue.

Obviously, your insulin levels are the lowest in the early morning hours before you wake because you are not eating anything during the overnight fast. More specifically, your insulin levels fall to baseline three to four hours after your last meal, or snack. They remain at the baseline (low) until you break your fast, commonly known as *breakfast*. If, like many people, you have an evening snack after dinner, say 9pm, your insulin levels will be at baseline from about midnight to six, or approximately six hours. During those six hours, while sleeping, you are burning fat, unless you break the fast early.

Unfortunately, even a low-carb snack containing protein or sugar-alcohol will cause a release of insulin. The effect is variable and may range from 40-60% of the amount you would see with white bread. Most foods, other than pure fat or celery or similar, will cause the release of insulin; therefore, the only way to keep your insulin levels at baseline is by not eating anything but fat or celery, and only a little celery.

Remember. Nighttime is good, especially if you avoid a nighttime snack and don't eat a glazed donut in the middle of it.

Conclusion #5

YOU ARE BEING OUTSMARTED BY A FEW STRANDS OF MICROSOPIC DNA FROM THE TIME OF DINOSAURS

You know what artificial intelligence is (AI). It's complex computer code that runs in the background to make choices and selections in algorithms to reach a result, like *Siri* of Apple or *Alexa* of Amazon. They are forms of AI. That's kind of what your DNA is, except that it's not artificial. It's biological. Call it "BI" for biological intelligence. Each and every one of your cells is packed with loads of DNA, BI, and it is operating in the background, making choices and selections based on the material presented to it.

Just as you can get Siri or Alexa to tell or say what you want by asking the right questions, so can you get your DNA, your biological intelligence, to do what you want, relative to weight-loss, by presenting it with the right materials (food energy), in the right order.

When I talk about good calories and bad calories, I am talking about the effects that some calories exert on your body's ability to burn and store fat, effects that some calories do better than others

It is your BI that rules the day when it comes to your body's ability to burn and store fat. It is quite beyond your control, unless you specifically control the material, in this case food, presented to your DNA. It is your DNA that decides what calories are good and what calories are bad, and although every calorie counts in a mechanical, perfect, bomb calorimeter; in you, the imperfect bomb calorimeter that you are, with all your hormones, enzymes and DNA, the brutal truth is that *some calories count more than others.*

DNA STRAND
Discovered by Watson and Crick in 1953.

Now, let us do a little thought experiment. We'll do another one a little later that is much more intricate. Thought experiments are cool, that's how Einstein derived his theory of relativity. He thought it, because there was no way to prove it until three decades more of technological advancement.

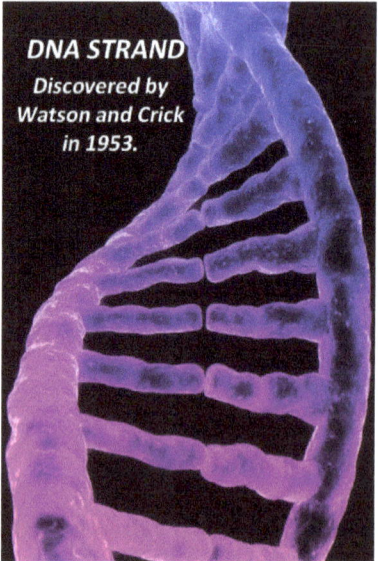

Let us imagine that we are in a contest with our DNA to store fat. The DNA wants to store fat, so the organism doesn't starve. You want to not store fat, so you lose weight.

Imagine this. You have a basal caloric requirement of 2000 calories to maintain your current weight. Imagine that you eat only fat, one pound of butter (four sticks a day) breakfast, lunch and dinner and a snack. One pound of butter contains about 3200 calories. Will you gain weight by storing the extra 1200 calories per day as fat, gaining one pound of fat every three days?

In my thought experiment, the answer is No. You will not, and you know why already. Does fat cause the release of insulin? No. What does insulin do? It builds up fat. When insulin levels are low, fat is being metabolized for energy needs (torn down). The environment inside your body is not favorable towards fat-storage. The DNA is frustrated, it wants insulin, but it has to follow the program. You will metabolize the fat, break it down, use it as energy, probably make a little glycogen, maybe even store a little fat here and there, but not much, and you will feel full because *fat is satiating*. It fills you up. You'll likely be full after the first stick. You would need to force yourself to eat the full pound.

> When **INSULIN LEVELS** are **LOW** in the blood stream the ENVIRONMENT for **FAT** storage is **POOR**.

Now, imagine this: The same caloric needs, but now you eat only sugar, two pounds of sugar in cherry Kool-Aide divided into four doses daily. Two pounds sugar equals about 3500 calories, not too dissimilar from your one pound of fat regimen. Will you gain weight by storing the extra 1500 calories as fat, gaining over a pound of fat every three days?

In my thought experiment, the answer is *you bet*, and you know this already as well. Does sugar cause the release of insulin? *You bet*. Lots of it. What does insulin do? *It makes fat*. The environment inside your body is very favorable towards fat-storage. Since you are on a two-pound sugar diet daily, your glycogen stores are already chock full so all those extra 1500 calories/day will move directly to fat storage. The DNA wins. Fat is beautiful. Your body rejoices. It will not starve. In fact, it's so good, you want more because *carbohydrates make you hungry*.

> When **INSULIN LEVELS** are **HIGH** in the blood stream the ENVIRONMENT for **FAT** storage is **EXCELLENT**.

Lastly, imagine this. Imagine that you're not sure if you prefer butter or sugar and so you eat half of both; half-a-pound of butter (two sticks) and one-pound of sugar a day. That equals 3400 calories, again, similar to the above. Will you gain weight by storing the extra 1400 calories per day, as fat, gaining over one pound of fat every three days?

In my thought experiment, the answer is *you bet*. Does the fat cause the release of insulin? No. Does the pound of sugar cause the release of insulin? You bet. What does insulin do?

Is there as much insulin in the blood stream with one pound of sugar as there is with two? Of course not. Logically, it's about half as much, but half as much is still more than plenty. As before, your glycogen stores are full, and all those extra calories move directly to fat storage. The DNA wins again. Fat is beautiful. You're going to live. When's dinner?

> With significant levels of insulin in the blood, *any amount of excess calories* (ingested fat has the most at 9Cal/gm.) will be turned into fat. To counter this, you must keep insulin levels low for at least parts of the day and night.

Can we stop this now? Do you better understand the biological intelligence inside your cells, and how it rules your body by following an instructional code that is millions of years old?

When you think about it, in the evolutionary sense, it is in fact very logical. Approximately 65 million years ago, about the time of the extinction-event that wiped out the dinosaurs, an asteroid strike it is thought, our two-foot tall ancestor (if it stood) not too dissimilar to a rat, poked it's long pointy nose out of a hole in the ground, in search of food, like insects, nuts and berries. It secreted insulin too.

Ardipithecus kadabba, one of the earliest known hominids, knocked about the African bush about 60 million years later, or about 5 million years ago, also eating nuts and berries and bugs, and probably rats too. (3) It also secreted insulin, in fact, the same or very similar to the molecular formula that is secreted by the beta cells of your pancreas today, or that which is injected by millions of people world-wide suffering from diabetes.

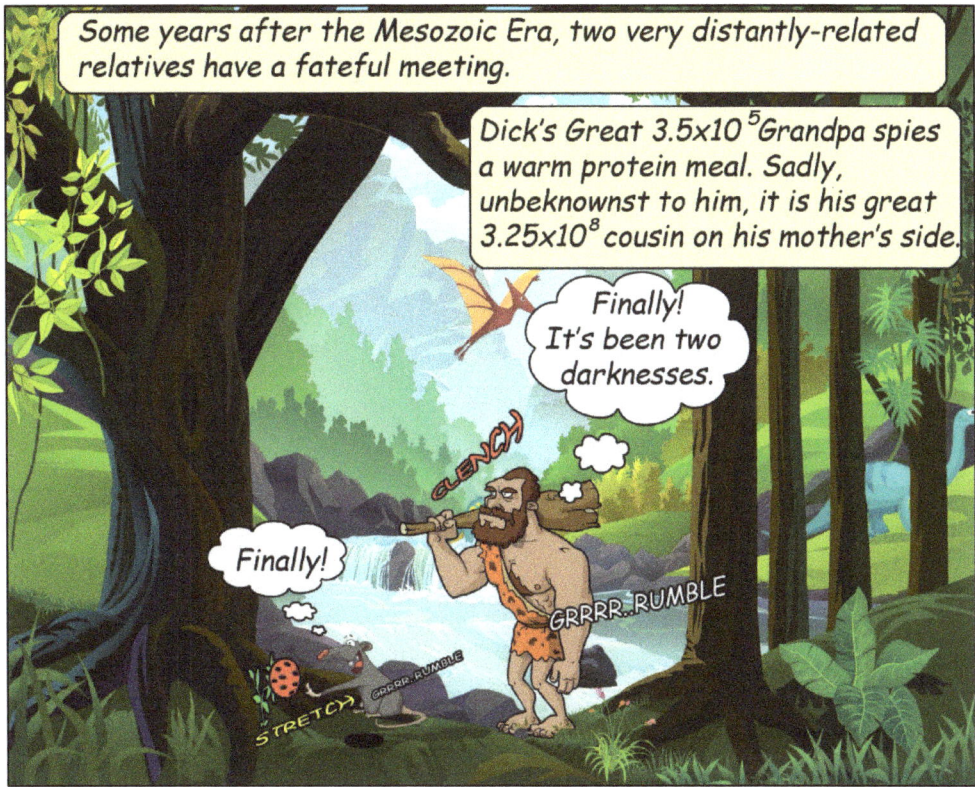

Do you think Ardipithecus had a bedtime snack or three squares a day? Of course not. When they had food they ate, when they didn't, they didn't. Our evolutionary reality is that we are built for feast and famine. It's like we were made to fast because if we couldn't, we would have died. Fasting is natural. Fasting is safe, if done appropriately. Fasting is harder for some than it is for others, at first. It gets easier.

So far, you have learned some biological truths, and have drawn some simplistic conclusions; now, it's time to apply your newfound knowledge. It is time for some *strategery*. It is my wish for you that the way you think about food and energy are changing. The truth is a powerful force. You are getting smarter, green belt even, the first arrow is nearly completely within your grasp.

Strategery #1

LIMIT YOUR CARBOHYDRATE INTAKE TO LESS THAN 100 GM/DAY (LOW -GLYCEMIC).

Glycemic Index (GI) is a measure of how quickly a food causes your blood sugar to rise.
A GI < 55 is better. A GI > 70 is bad.

When you limit your carbohydrate intake, you are in effect managing your insulin levels by limiting the levels of insulin that are released into the bloodstream after ingesting carbohydrates. By eating lower glycemic carbohydrates, and fewer carbohydrates, you decrease the amount of insulin released and it is released slower than it would be otherwise with the ingestion of sugar or high-glycemic carbs.

This is not draconian at all (100gm/day). You do have to count, and it does add up in a hurry. For instance the two slices of a whole-wheat bread on either side of ham and cheese will have nearly 50 grams of carbohydrate, unless they're one of the lower-carb slices, which only means that it's a smaller and thinner slice of bread, almost like a soft cracker it seems.

When you count carbs, subtract the grams of fiber because it doesn't represent sugar. For instance, in the one slice of whole wheat bread there are 24 grams of carbohydrate and 3 grams of fiber; therefore, I count 21 net grams of carbohydrate.

If you're not eating as many carbs, that means you'll be eating more protein and fat, which as fine, if the sources are good: lean meats (grass-fed), dairy, eggs, cheese, poultry, fish, vegetables.

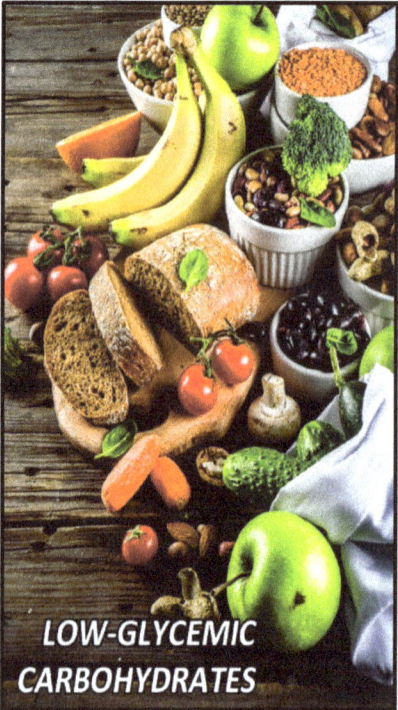

LOW-GLYCEMIC CARBOHYDRATES

Generally, fruit is discouraged, if your objective is losing weight as it is higher carb, even if natural and lower-glycemic.

As I have mentioned previously, my bias is towards the low-carb, ketogenic spectrum, and this strategy is specific to it; however, most conventional, caloric restricted diets do pay homage to some form of carbohydrate control, if only towards the avoidance of sugar, refined carbohydrates and similar high-glycemic carbs that cause quicker and higher surges of insulin release into the blood.

The advantage of restricting carbohydrates is that you thereby suppress the release of insulin, and you now know that if you suppress insulin you by default *suppress the suppression* of fat metabolism. *Did you get that, the double negative?* It's good.

If there is little or no sugar (carbohydrate) in the blood, there is little or minimal insulin, which means that when at rest, your body is pretty much forced to burn fat for ongoing energy needs. If you are exerting yourself, your body will metabolize your glycogen stores first before resorting to fat stores. I realize that I'm saying the same thing over and over in slightly different ways, but it's important. If you eat carbs, you burn carbs for energy, and whatever you don't immediately use gets turned into glycogen and then into fat. If you don't eat many carbs, you burn mostly fat for energy. This is why low-carb diets are so popular, because they work well for most people. On a low-carb diet, your glycogen stores will be at least partially depleted, and you will preferentially metabolize fat for basal metabolic needs throughout the day between meals *if you don't snack*, and of course, also during the nighttime *if you don't keep a box of donuts on the nightstand.*

Now we're going to take it up a notch. You're going to learn how to manage your insulin levels like a Zen master.

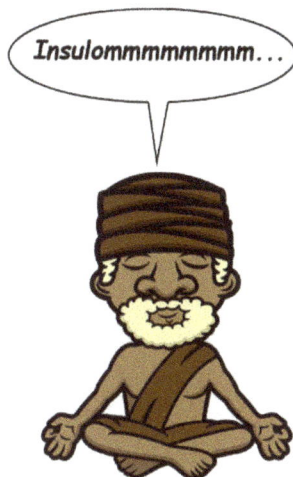

Strategery #2

EXTEND YOUR OVERNIGHT FAST. A **12H** FAST.

Not eating after dinner equates to about a twelve-hour fast, which means your insulin levels would be baseline for about *nine hours* of definite fat burning.

A 12H fast is as simple as not eating after dinner, until breakfast. No nighttime snacks.

The most natural way to prolong the low-insulin, fat-metabolizing state is to extend the overnight fast. This could be done in two stages as *fasting* might sound scary. It did to me, and I immediately discounted it until completing further research. Initially, I had the conviction that fasting would lower my metabolic rate, which was wrong. It does not. In fact, it increases it. It is only after three days of fasting that your basal metabolic rate begins to drop, for example, if you are floating in a dingy on the ocean after your boat sunk and have run out of food (4).

A severe caloric restriction (VLCD) beyond a few days will lower you Basal Metabolic Rate. Intermittent Fasting *does not*.

What does lower your metabolic rate is a very low-calorie diet (VLCD), day after day, because that little bit of glandular tissue at the base of the brain interprets that as *starving*, and then things slow down (5). This is why those VLCD of less than 1000 Calories per day, usually eaten through a straw, are counterproductive. Oh, you lose weight, that's for sure, if you are compliant, but as soon as you begin eating normally, which everyone eventually does, the weight pours back on because your basal metabolic rate (BMR) was reset to a lower value since you were *starving*. Whether or not your BMR ever returns to your pre-VLCD level is debatable and multifactorial. It is not black and white. There is far more nuance than everything I have shared with you thus far. If you are interested in the nuance, I have posted a further in-depth explanation on my website, *FatThief.com*.

Strategery #3

EXTEND YOUR OVERNIGHT FAST MORE. AN **18H** FAST.

This is what I'm currently doing. I don't eat after dinner and skip breakfast; so, I eat lunch and dinner between 12 and 6 pm, which means that I fast eighteen

An 18H fast is as easy as not eating after dinner and skipping breakfast.

hours every day. Sometimes I have a snack in the afternoon, but usually not because I'm not hungry, and besides, why break that intermittent fast of the intermittent fast, which amounts to a couple of more hours of fat metabolism.

The strategy of intermittent fasting *is a functional strategy*, it is not a religious one. If you break the fast, you won't go to hell. There will be times, special occasions, like weddings or a birthday party or Thanksgiving, during which you will not fast, but during those times you will eat mostly sensibly, and when the occasion is over, you revert to your normal, or *new normal* I should say.

In the mornings, I do drink coffee with a coconut oil powder additive that also has some artificial sweetener. I buy it from Costco.com. I like it. I also have a large glass of water with Benefiber and two fiber gummy cubes. That is my breakfast and it is not a strict fast, but the fat of the coconut oil does cause some measure of satiety that easily carries me to lunch or beyond. The coffee and creamer will cause a slight rise in insulin w/some suppression of fat metabolism, but it is my view that it is of questionable significance against the backdrop of an 18H fast.

The hardest time for me is at night. If I stay up later, I get hungry, but I acknowledge that, and sometimes I have to whip out my second or third arrow. It gets easier.

KETOGENIC diets require a *severe restriction in carbohydrates* to **less than 50 gms./day**. The glycogen stores are exhausted, and the body is forced to burn fat as a primary energy source. **KETONE BODIES** are produced when the fat is burned and are used as an energy source.

A true ketogenic diet is very difficult for some people beyond a few days as it excludes significant amounts of sweet potatoes, squash, whole grains, fruits, and many other otherwise healthy foods that make excellent side dishes. On the other hand, because of the forced fat metabolism, the ketogenic diet is quite effective in the lessening of fat stores. For me, I find it more difficult than intermittent fasting, which I view as an alternative way to managing your insulin levels in order to enhance fat metabolism. In fact, I combine low-carb, if not strictly ketogenic, with intermittent fasting, and by this I mean to say 100-150gm of carbs/day.

In a strict ketogenic diet, your glycogen stores are chronically depleted, so the body's primary choice for energy becomes the fat stores because the glycogen bucket is empty, even if there is a significant amount of insulin in the blood from the protein portion of your diet of three squares a day, plus all those snacks of beef jerky, pickled turkey gizzards, pigs feet and hard-boiled eggs.

In an intermittent fasting strategy, your glycogen stores are at least partially full, but you metabolize fat directly from the fat bucket because that is what the body does for the six or 12 or 18 or whatever hours there are low insulin levels in your blood stream. *Remember, it takes roughly three hours for the insulin levels to fall to baseline after a meal or snack.*

Please note the caution, action item. I made it to look like a chainsaw because I am totally serious. If you are taking medication (especially insulin) and begin a strict ketogenic or low-carb diet, you can get in serious trouble, much more so than you can with a chainsaw.

IF YOU EMBARK UPON A TRUE KETOGENIC DIET, PLEASE DO SO UNDER THE GUIDANCE OF YOUR HEALTHCARE PROVIDER, ESPECIALLY IF TAKING MEDICATIONS.

Remember. We are imperfect bomb calorimeters. Of course, the relationship between the increase in insulin and the corresponding decrease in fat metabolism is not perfectly symmetrical. The purpose of the graph in Figure C is simply to provide a visual representation of the metabolic consequences of ingesting the macronutrients. The important part is the *area under the curve* and how we might modify that to our advantage. It should be obvious, also, based on what has been covered thus far, that the area under the curve will be increased (higher peaks, shallower valleys, longer duration) with the ingestion of sugar (soda, sweets, high fructose corn syrup in low-fat products, etc.) and refined carbohydrates (soft white stuff, etc.).

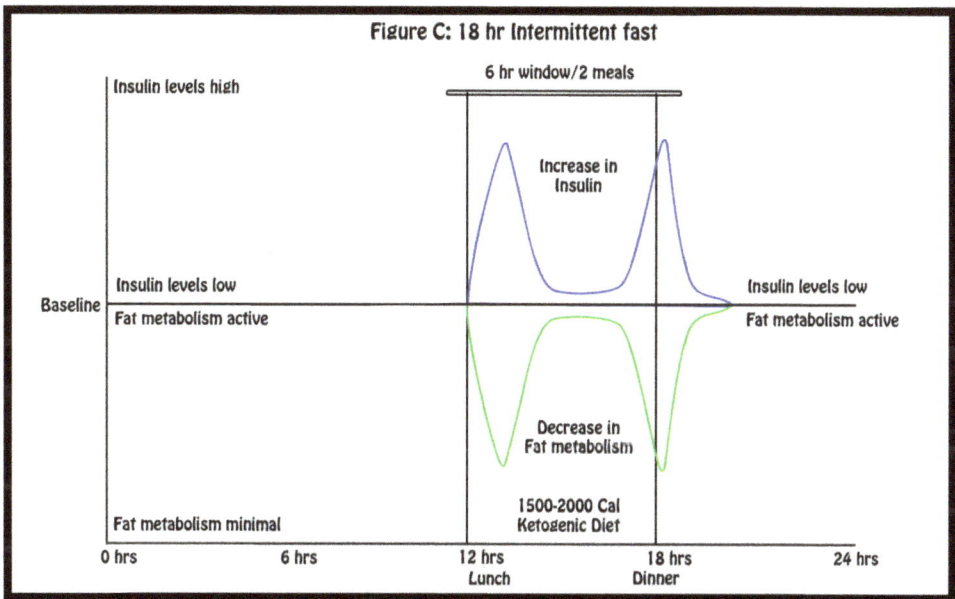

Figure C: 18 hr Intermittent fast

6 hr window/2 meals

Insulin levels high

Increase in Insulin

Baseline

Insulin levels low
Fat metabolism active

Insulin levels low
Fat metabolism active

Decrease in Fat metabolism

1500-2000 Cal Ketogenic Diet

Fat metabolism minimal

| 0 hrs | 6 hrs | 12 hrs | 18 hrs | 24 hrs |
| | | Lunch | Dinner | |

The GOAL of INTERMITTENT FASTING is to decrease the **total amount of and time of** exposure to INSULIN in the blood stream.

This is accomplished be eating less frequently (two times in Fig. C) and no snacking between meals.

Now, for the sake of comparison, let us consider the graphical representation of the typical American diet (TAD) which we saw in a previous illustration. This might not be too much different from what you are presently doing. I used to do this, because I felt there was a metabolic benefit to eating every 3-4 hours. There is not. There is a slight increase in metabolism, up to 25% of the caloric content of the food, called *Diet Induced Thermogenesis (DIT)*; however, this response is blunted in overweight individuals (6) and any minimal gain is likely more than offset by the decrease in fat metabolism due to the insulin induced suppression.

In the TAD, with three meals, and snacks between meals and in the evening, there is minimal fat metabolism during waking hours because your body preferentially burns carbohydrates, and then glycogen. If your diet is low-carb or ketogenic, then you will have minimal circulating carbs and depleted glycogen stores, and you *will* still metabolize fat; however, the TAD *is not* ketogenic and, sadly, there is suppression of fat metabolism all through the day and into the night. In Figure D, below, pay attention to the area under the curve.

Consider the amount of bad fats, sugar, soft white stuff and high fructose corn syrup in the TAD. Is it any wonder that we are suffering an epidemic of obesity?

> The Typical American Diet does not allow for fat burning during waking hours and into the night because of frequent eating.

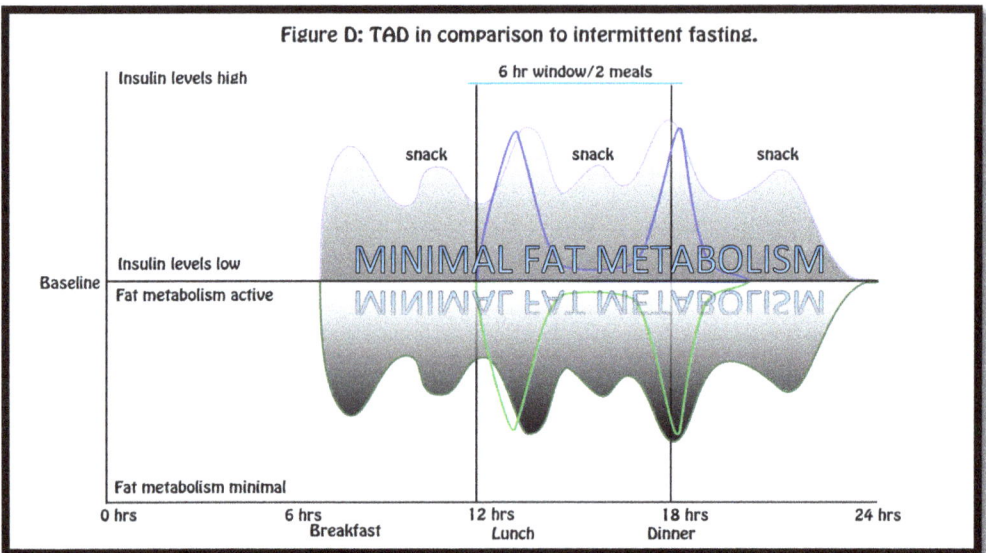

Figure D: TAD in comparison to intermittent fasting.

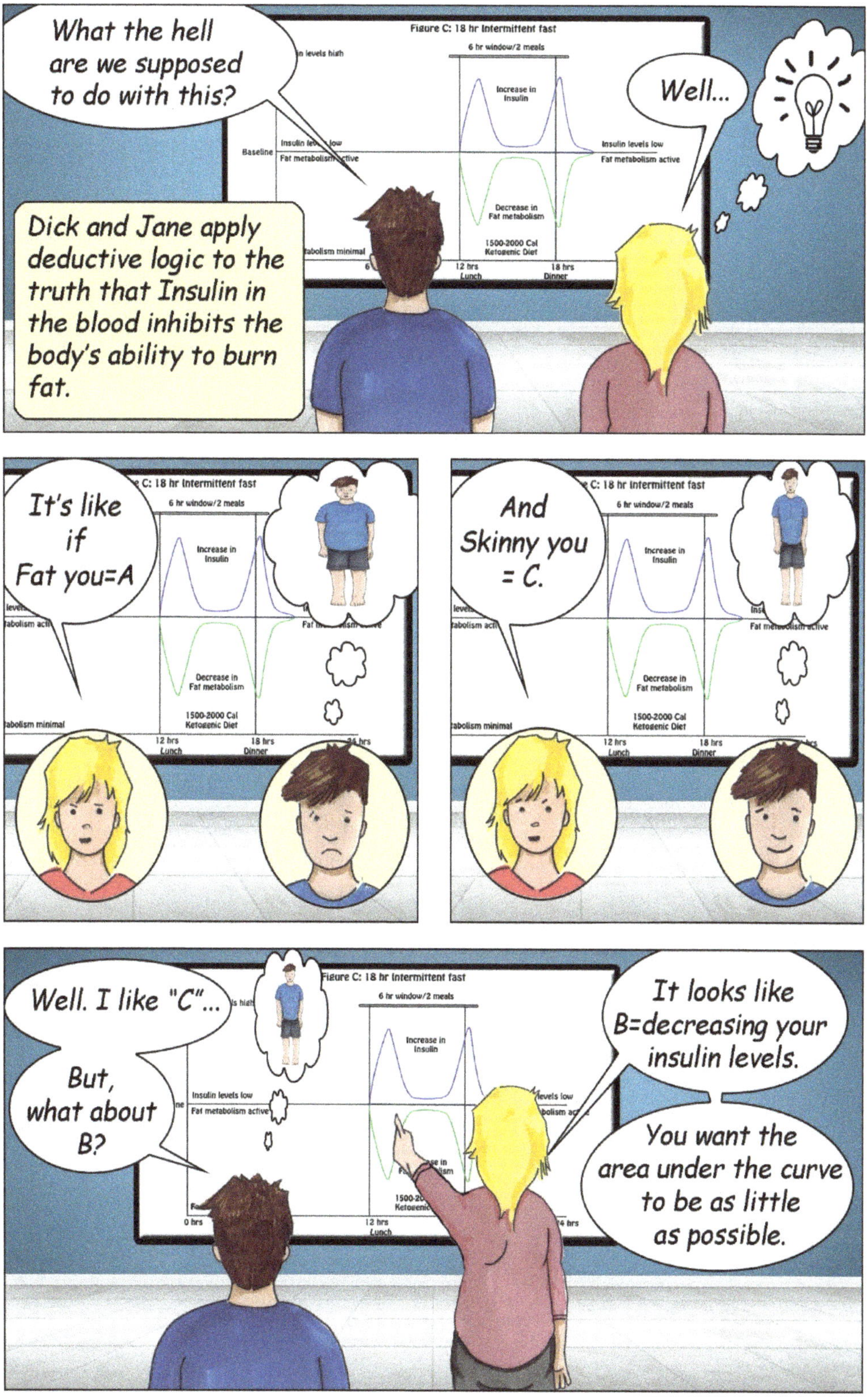
What the hell are we supposed to do with this?
Figure C: 18 hr Intermittent fast
6 hr window/2 meals
Increase in Insulin
Insulin levels low
Fat metabolism active
Decrease in Fat metabolism
1500-2000 Cal Ketogenic Diet
12 hrs Lunch
18 hrs Dinner
Well...
Dick and Jane apply deductive logic to the truth that Insulin in the blood inhibits the body's ability to burn fat.
It's like if Fat you=A
And Skinny you = C.
Well. I like "C"...
But, what about B?
It looks like B=decreasing your insulin levels.
You want the area under the curve to be as little as possible.

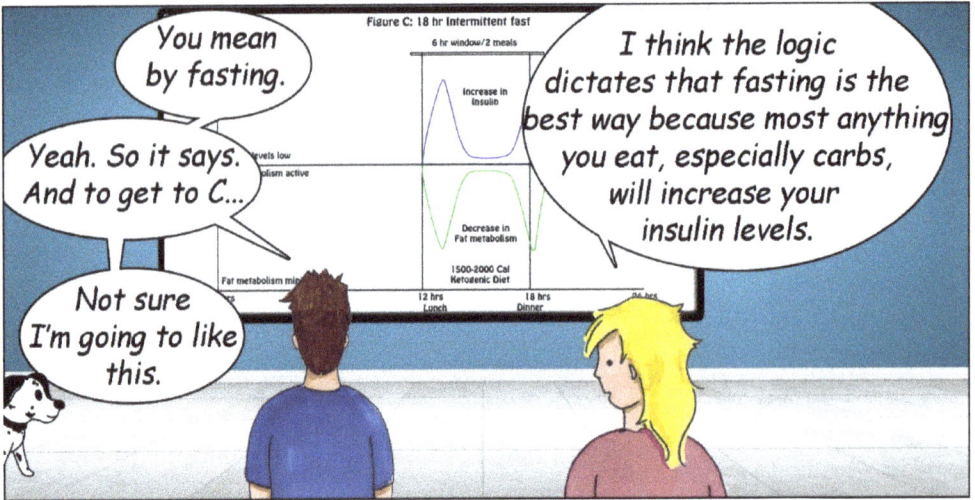

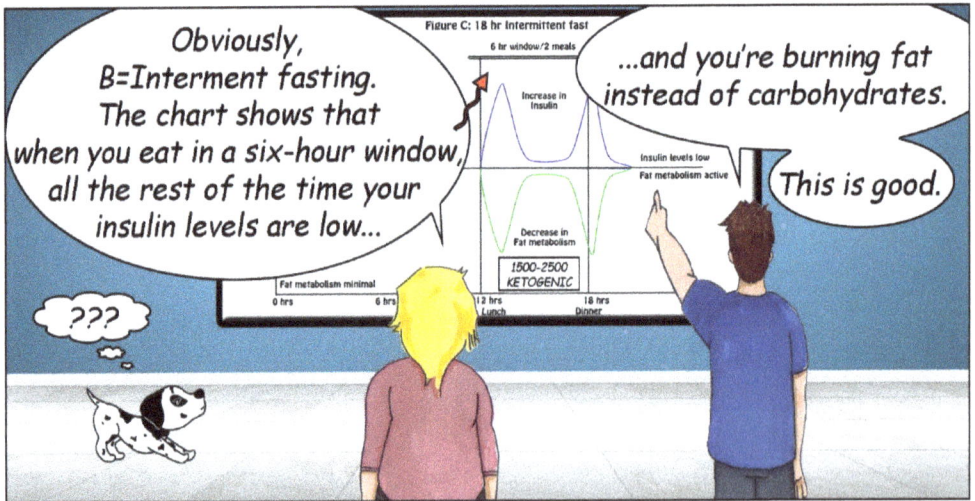

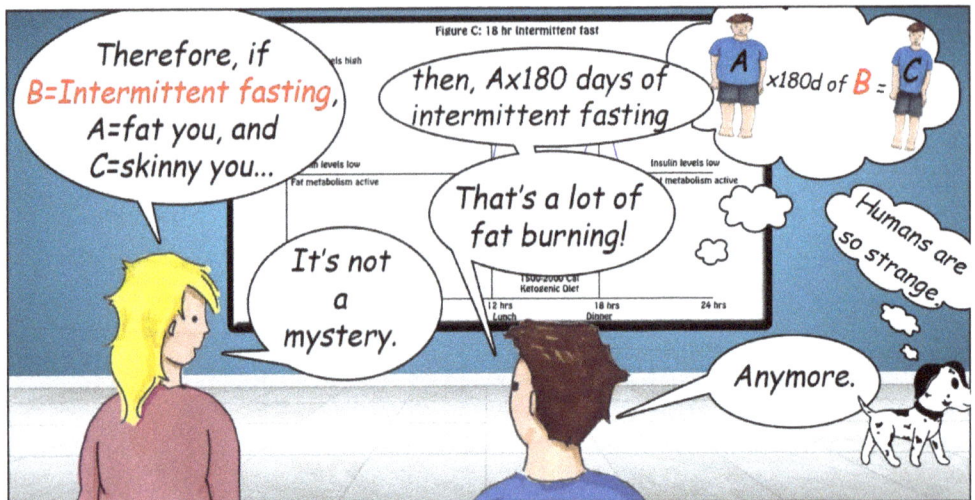

Strategery #4

FAST LIKE YOU'RE CRAZY, BUT NOT LONGER THAN THREE DAYS.

There are many intermittent fasting regimens, including fasts measured in days rather than hours. Fasting for more than 24 is more aggressive and definitely not for someone of questionable health or who is on medications. I might consider trying a two to three day fast someday if my wife visits her mother in North Dakota because that means I wouldn't have to clean up after myself in the kitchen (which I always do of course) so if I don't eat, no mess. Easy-peazy.

I take that back. During the several month process of editing, my wife did leave town for a few days, and I couldn't do it. Not easy-peazy for me. I didn't see the point really as I've already had tremendous success with my 18hr intermittent fast. I would further note that a close acquaintance has had equal success with a low-carb diet (<150gm/day) combined with a 12hr intermittent fast.

The advantage to a longer fast is a longer period of time free from the effects of insulin. The longest documented fast was 382 days in which a 27-year-old man went from 456 pounds to 180 pounds (7). This was a medically supervised fast in Scotland, in the 1970s.

There are several different intermittent fasting regimens; 12H, 18H, 24h, 36h, alternate days--there may be a point where you might plateau in which case something should change. Our bodies are masters of adaptation; therefore, variety and change are good.

There are many different ways to combine strategies (caloric control/carb control/intermittent fasting).

There are many different fasting periods, both in length (12-36hr.) and in time of day, if necessary (i.e. working night-time shift).

We are almost done with phase III. I have told you the truth. It should be completely clear how your body responds to carbohydrates, fat and protein, and the role insulin plays. If there remains some cloudiness, please page through and review all the key points in bold and in the text boxes.

There are many more chemical mediators and hormones and enzymes, but these truths I have shared with you are the most important and if you respect them, they will work to your advantage.

The Seven Biological Truths
1. INSULIN TURNS OFF FAT METABOLISM AND STORES ENERGY (FOOD) AS FAT OR GLYCOGEN.
2. CARBOHYDRATE/SUGAR IS THE PRIMARY MACRONUTRIENT THAT CAUSES THE RELEASE OF INSULIN.
3. PROTEIN ALSO CAUSES THE RELEASE OF INSULIN, NOT AS MUCH AS CARBOHYDRATES, BUT IT STILL DOES.
4. FAT IS STORED ENERGY. IT DOES NOT CAUSE A SIGNIFICANT RELEASE OF INSULIN IF INGESTED.
5. GLYCOGEN IS STORED ENERGY. IT IS THE STORAGE FORM OF CARBOHYDRATE/GLUCOSE.
6. INSULIN TURNS NEARLY ALL INGESTED FOOD NOT USED FOR METABOLIC NEEDS INTO GLUCOSE THEN INTO GLYCOGEN THEN INTO FAT, IN THAT ORDER.
7. YOUR BODY WILL ALWAYS BURN GLUCOSE OR GLYCOGEN FIRST, WHEN GIVEN THE CHOICE.

REMEMBER TO REFER TO APPENDICES FOR SUMMATION LISTS AND HOW TO REFERENCES.

THE FINAL TRUTH

OBESITY KILLS.

The final truth in Phase III you must appreciate is that obesity will kill you. This is the tip of the spear, or rather, the sharp point of the arrow relative to this arrow of truth. It is what caused me to write down this manual before you, because, when I thought I was dying and the only thing I could do to potentially keep that from happening was to change the way I ate, it all became easy. I thought I might possibly make it as easy for others too.

On October 24ᵗʰ, 2018, a Wednesday morning, I woke up with a deep vibration in my right chest. It felt like a bad subwoofer, buzzing with each breath. I immediately recognized it, because I had a similar condition 15 years earlier that affected the pericardium, which is the sac that surrounds the heart. I knew that this time it was the pleura, which is the lining of the lungs, which is simply a continuation of the same layer of the pericardium. Fifteen years ago, I had my pericardium surgically removed at the Mayo Clinic. I knew that there was not a similar surgical option with the pleura.

I texted a friend I worked with who was a pulmonologist.

"Hi Rich. I have a right pleural rub. No pain, just awareness of it. Should I just give it a few days? Sorry to hit you up like this. Ur snake-bit friend."

Before I texted, I stood in my closet with my stethoscope held to my right side. I heard the classic rub that is described as the sound of leather on leather, from the friction of the parietal pleura (lining inside of chest wall) rubbing against the visceral pleura (lining around lung). I signed off as "ur snake-bit friend," because that's how Rich often referred to patients in difficult situations where things weren't going right: "They're snake-bit," he'd say.

A few days later, a chest CT confirmed a bilateral pleuritis, worse on the right, with calcifications suggesting chronicity. That night, I researched bilateral fibrosing pleuritis. It wasn't good. I felt my grip on this mortal coil loosening. I was sitting upstairs in my home office. I heard my wife downstairs in the kitchen. I wondered what I was going to do, what I could do. I remembered reading Paul Kalanithi's *When Breath Becomes Air*, and I thought, this is too important to not record in some fashion, to somehow communicate to others the preciousness that each breath is. Then I had an idea. I thought I would write an anonymous blog. I went to my GoDaddy account and searched *TheDyingMan.com*.

Can you believe it? It was available. I still haven't told anyone about it other than some close friends and a few cousins. It's a chronicle of that whole experience.

The problem with obesity is that the fat, which is called White Adipose Tissue (**WAT**), is not a chemically inert padding making smooth edges from sharp ones, or soft surfaces of hard ones; it is chemically active, like a gland, but what it secretes is not good. Like the thyroid secretes thyroxin, or the adrenal epinephrine, or the pancreatic beta cells insulin; the WAT secretes some really very bad stuff. In the spirit of gross simplification, the WAT secretes multiple chemical mediators that cause a low-grade inflammation throughout the body. In medicine we call this a *systemic* process because it involves all the organ systems, and why wouldn't it? It's in the blood after all. (8)

Chronic inflammation is at the root of many disease processes such as Lupus, Rheumatoid Arthritis, Ulcerative Colitis, Crohn's Disease. It is the chronic inflammation in the lining of the coronary arteries that lead to plaque build-up and occlusion and heart disease, as is the case with the aorta and the arteries to the extremities and to the brain. This is just one example of obesity-related inflammation--the systemic effect it exerts on the vascular system. That is what obesity does. It leads to a pro-inflammatory state, which leads to the metabolic syndrome, and all the other really very bad stuff.

I have described the chronic inflammatory condition that I suffered, which precipitated this effort. I had a chronic inflammatory condition, bilateral fibrosing pleuritis, for which the endpoint was progression, and all I could do to halt that progression, other than anti-inflammatory medications, was to interrupt the condition of inflammation by diet, and by decreasing the volume of my WAT *gland*.

It is not a question of if. It is a question of when. It is a certainty that an obese individual, and especially a morbidly obese individual, will live less well and live less long than one who is not. The scariest of all the inflammatory-related effects of obesity are the obesity-related cancers for they are of course, in many cases, a potential near-term terminal event.

Do you feel smarter? You should. This is a tremendous amount of very important information. I want for you to do well and to be successful. You are the reason. Congratulations. I hereby promote you to *Brown-belt* in the Obesity-dragon slaying class.

REVIEW THE REMAINING PAGES IN THIS CHAPTER FOR LISTS OF OBESITY-RELATED DISEASE AND A COMPLETE SUMMARY OF ACTIONS TO TAKE.

The Really Very Bad Stuff (9)

OBESITY RELATED ILLNESS

1. HIGH BLOOD PRESSURE
2. HIGH LDL (BAD CHOLESTEROL)
3. TYPE 2 DIABETES
4. NONALCOHOLIC STEATOHEPATITIS (NASH)
5. CORONARY HEART DISEASE
6. STROKE
7. GALLBLADDER DISEASE
8. OSTEOARTHRITIS
9. SLEEP APNEA
10. MENTAL ILLNESS
11. IMPAIRED PHYSICAL FUNCTIONING

OBESITY RELATED CANCERS

1. BREAST, AFTER MENOPAUSE
2. COLON AND RECTUM
3. ENDOMETRIAL (UTERINE)
4. GALLBLADDER
5. KIDNEY
6. LIVER
7. ESOPHAGEAL
8. STOMACH
9. PANCREATIC
10. OVARIAN
11. MULTIPLE MYELOMA
12. KIDNEY

*White Adipose Tissue (**WAT**) in the obese can act like a gland by secreting (releasing) harmful chemicals in the blood stream.
*The WAT that is above the waist and inside the abdomen, around and in the organs, is especially noted for the secretion of pro-inflammatory mediators.

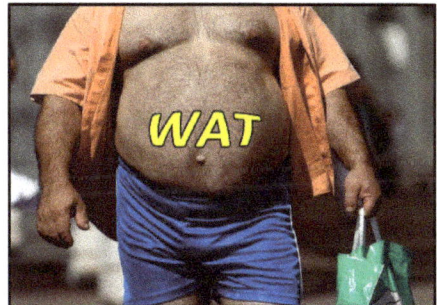

WAT is also associated with the Metabolic Syndrome that is the precursor to and associated with many illnesses, including diabetes.

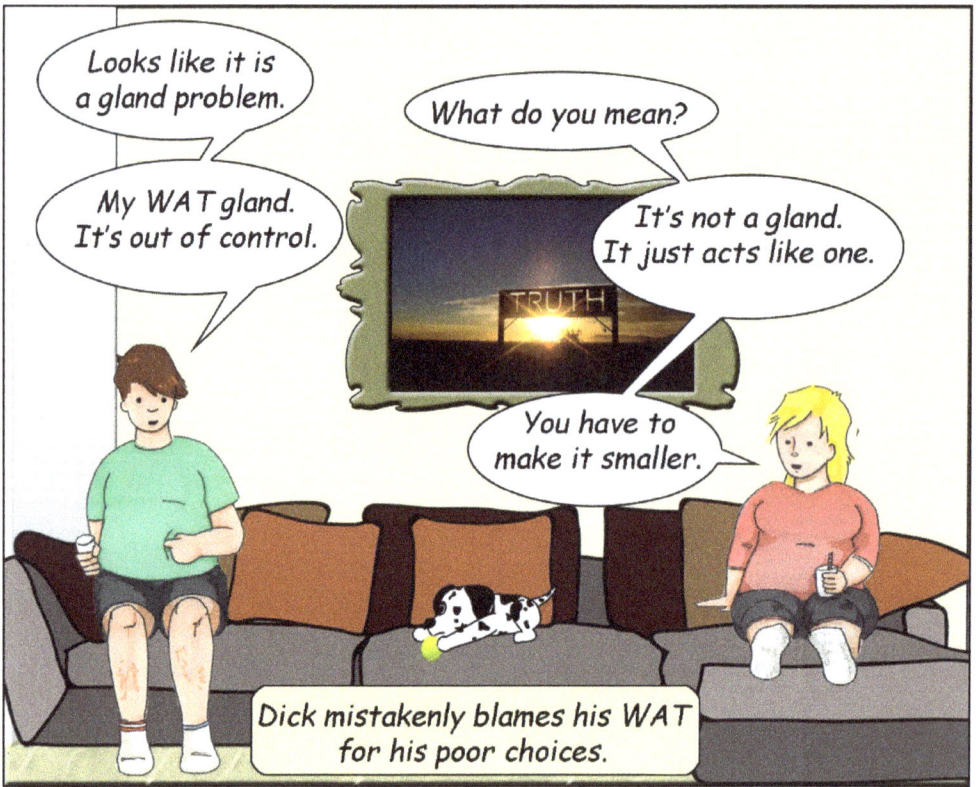

Dick mistakenly blames his WAT for his poor choices.

YOU ARE SEEING FREQUENT REFERENCES TO THE APPENDICES. YOU MAY REFER TO THESE AT ANYTIME, HOWEVER THE PRIMARY FUNCTION OF THE APPENDICES IS FOR **AFTER** YOU FINISH THE BOOK AND VIDEOS BECAUSE THE APPENDICES REPRESENT YOUR TASKS AND CHECKLISTS IN THE SPECIFIC ORDER YOU SHOULD COMPLETE THEM.

In Summary

1. PICK A DIET PLAN: MY BIAS IS TOWARDS A LOW-CARB KETOGENIC, ANTI-INFLAMMATORY STRATEGY. IT IS MY FEELING THAT THESE DIETS ARE EASIER TO COMPLY WITH AS THEY ARE LESS RESTRICTIVE THAN THE PLANT-BASED, ANIMAL-PRODUCT-AVOIDANCE STRATEGY; BUT, YOU'RE THE BOSS. PICK WHATEVER YOU WANT.

2. PREPARE YOUR CASTLE: MAKE YOUR HOME A SAFE PLACE. IT IS YOUR FORTRESS OF SOLITUDE THAT SHOULD BE IMPERVIOUS TO THE DRAGON. HAVE A STRATEGY FOR HOW YOU'RE GOING TO EAT WHEN OUTSIDE THE WALL.

3. USE AN ONLINE BASAL CALORIC NEED CALCULATOR TO FIGURE OUT HOW MANY CALORIES YOU SHOULD CONSUME PER DAY TO LOSE 1-2 POUNDS PER WEEK: IF YOU ARE ON ONE OF THE DIETS TOWARDS EITHER EXTREME OF LOW-FAT, PLANT-BASED; OR, LOW-CARB KETOGENIC, COUNTING CALORIES IS LESS IMPORTANT, BUT I THINK IT IS STILL HELPFUL FOR A FEW WEEKS, UNTIL YOU HAVE AN APPRECIATION OF HOW MANY CALORIES ARE IN THE FOODS YOU EAT. HTTPS://WWW.NIDDK.NIH.GOV/BWP

4. BE HONEST. BE TRUE TO YOURSELF. CONTROL WHAT YOU EAT.

5. UNDERSTAND THE EFFECT INSULIN HAS ON YOUR FAT METABOLISM: IT'S BAD. INSULIN MAKES FAT.

6. LIMIT YOUR CARBOHYDRATES TO LESS THAN 100 GRAMS/DAY: ZERO SUGAR OR REFINED CARBOHYDRATES.

7. IMPLEMENT AN INTERMITTENT FASTING STRATEGY: ALTERNATING DAYS OF FASTING, OR A DAILY 16-18 HOUR EXTENDED NIGHTTIME FAST.

8. UNDERSTAND THAT THE DRAGON OF OBESITY WILL KILL YOU: YOU WILL LIVE LESS, AND YOU WILL LIVE LESS WELL THAN YOU OTHERWISE WOULD.

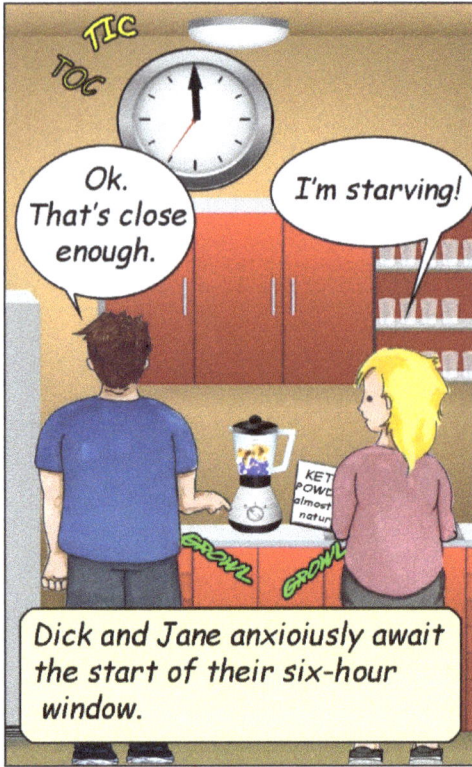

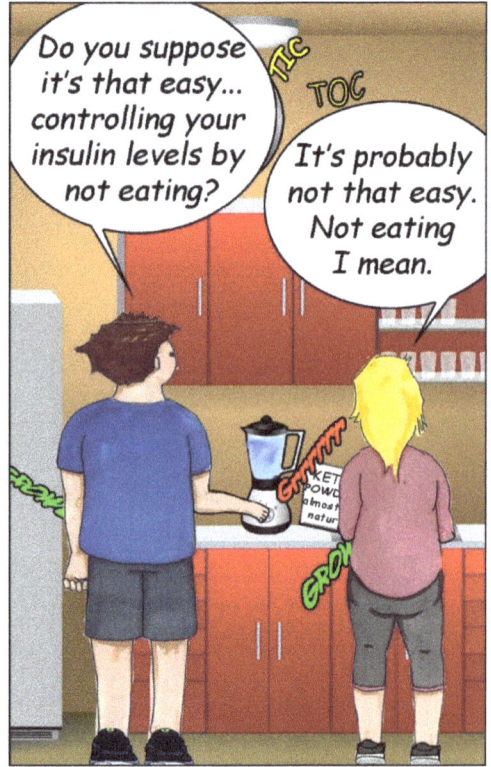

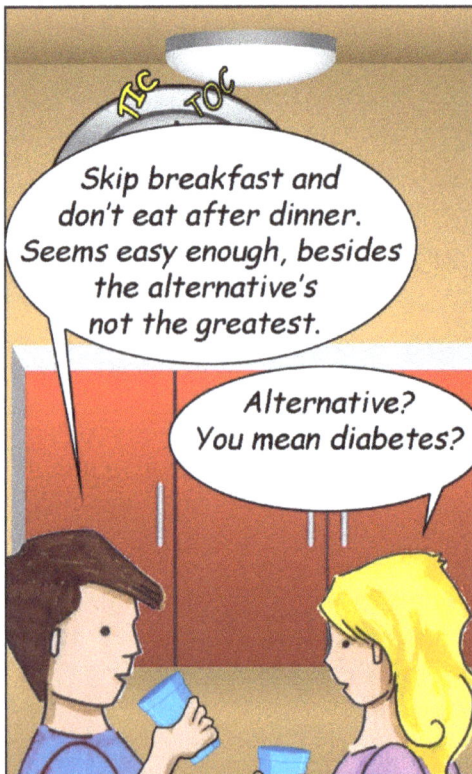

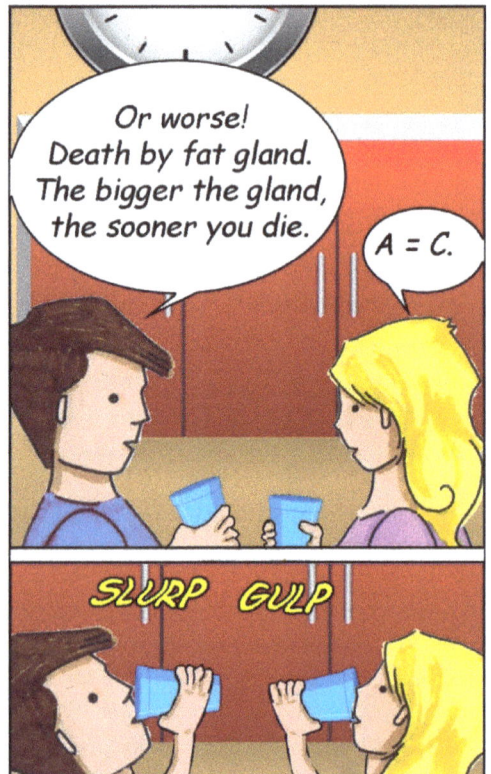

CHAPTER SIX: Phase IV: Exercise and Loose Ends

Phase IV:
1. Understand the truth about exercise.
2. Aerobic or Resistance or both?

You are not going to exercise your way to a normal BMI without also **not eating** your way to a normal BMI.

It is far easier to **not eat** your way towards a normal BMI than it is to exercise your way to a normal BMI.

S. J. Melarvie

The truth about exercise is that it is not that important, relative to your diet, for the primary goal of losing weight. This is due to the beautiful efficiency of how we were created: we accumulate and store massive amounts of energy easily, and we expend energy as efficiently, which is to say, hard. It is far easier to gain weight than it is to lose it, in other words. For this reason, it is a fallacy to propose that you can lose a significant amount of weight by exercise alone.

For example, assume an individual with a BMI of 35 (5'8", 230 lbs.) goes for a walk after dinner for one hour at a brisk pace of 4 MPH, which assumes a respectable baseline level of fitness. He or she would burn about 700 Calories. He or she would probably break a sweat and need to clean up or rest a bit prior to tackling some other task or pursuit, so there would be another twenty or so minutes of that on the back end, in total, estimate an hour-and-a-half time investment for one hour of moderately easy exercise, at least, to burn 700 calories.

How long does it take you to consume 700 calories? One of those 20 oz. bottles of Coke contain 248 calories. A 16 oz. *White Chocolate Mocha* from *Starbucks* contains 360 calories.

One case in which *losing weight by exercise alone* might apply is in the case of an otherwise healthy person who is overweight or mildly obese who changes not their diet, but decides to enter a marathon, or equivalent, and begins a serious training program. Even then, it is difficult to subtract out the diet because it is likely that part of that program involves healthier eating, as well as less time to eat.

This manual is for the obese, as I once was, and it is to those legions so afflicted that I owe my allegiance. Exercise is good and necessary, but it is like changing your socks: you should do it at least every other day, and it doesn't need to take all that much longer. Anything counts; walking to get the mail instead of using the Little Rascal, using the stairs instead of the elevator, picking weeds, filling the water softener, using a push mower instead of a rider, vacuuming the house.

For the obese, the more official types of exercise should be low impact, such as **walking or biking or swimming or equivalent. Twenty to thirty minutes every other day as a minimum** to start is not that much more time than it takes to change and launder your socks. It is likely that as your weight-loss progresses, it will become easier and more enjoyable as you become faster and stronger.

PLEASE REFER TO THE APPENDICES FOR SUPPLEMENTAL INFORMATION FOR EXERCISE RECOMMENDATIONS.

VISIT FATTHIEF.COM FOR HELPFUL LINKS.

Walking, jogging, bike riding, and swimming are all examples of aerobic exercise, which is good for the heart. The other side of the exercise equation is resistance training, which means weightlifting or using resistance bands, or exercises utilizing your own body weight, like pushups and pullups and leg squats.

It is often the case that resistance training is discounted, if not completely ignored, and this is wrong. Resistance training is equally important, if not more so, in my view, than aerobic training due to the age-related issue of lean body (muscle) loss. The naturally occurring loss of muscle mass with aging is called sarcopenia, and it is not desirable.

In a youngster of thirty, the lean muscle mass is about 50% of total body weight. Beginning about that time of relative youth there is a gradual loss of muscle mass down to 25% of total body weight by your 70s.

The age-related loss of muscle tissue is called SARCOPENIA. Between the ages of 30 and 70 you will lose half your muscle mass unless you exercise regularly, resistance training is very important in this regard.

To add insult to injury, the basal metabolic rate (BMR) declines as well since the lean body mass has a higher cost of metabolism than fat. This amounts to a 30% decrease in the BMR between the ages of 20 and 70. Bummer (10).

Sarcopenia. Sounds scary. It should be. It has the potential to turn you into a hunchbacked brittle old person that will fracture a thoracic vertebra with a vigorous sneeze. Sarcopenia is multifactorial of course, like everything else, and genetics is probably the strongest predicter, like everything else; however, if you are predisposed towards it, you will definitely get it and you will get it worse than you would if you don't take steps to address it. How do you not get sarcopenia? How do you not turn into a fragile, hump-backed bell-ringer with a heart of gold stumbling along on arthritic legs that sound like you're cracking nuts with each bend of the knee? Resistance training, of course. I would even go out on a limb and say that if you had to pick only one, between aerobic or resistance training, I'd pick resistance training. Definitely.

> The keys to exercise are that you enjoy it enough that you regularly do it, and that it also includes resistance training at least once a week, preferably twice.

My goal is to not turn you into a spandex-suited Marvel-worthy superhero rippling with muscle, although that is possible, and could follow. My goal is for you to lose weight in the most efficient way possible so that you may live longer and live better than you otherwise would. My exercise recommendations are not for the competitive athlete, they are for you. It is not so much important what you do as it is that *you do something*. It is helpful if it is something you halfway enjoy.

In my basement I have a treadmill, a recumbent bike and this thing called a Versa climber that is like a Stairmaster. I have **resistance bands** and a set of **adjustable dumbbells** for weights. This works for me. I do **resistance training for about 60 minutes once or twice a week** and aerobic training a similar amount. This is not a lot of exercise, but I also try to stay active outside. It is important for you to find what works for you. It may be a course of physical therapy prescribed by your primary care provider, or a **membership at the YMCA or other fitness facility**. Memberships in those facilities also allow access to personal trainers to get you started on an appropriate program.

If you are obese, and especially if you are morbidly obese or are taking prescription medications, all the above should be done with the permission and guidance of your primary care provider. They will assist you with the suitability of the exercise component to fit your needs.

Well, I didn't plan it this way, but my list turned out to be that divine number of 10, as in the Ten Commandments. We have applied seven biological truths in a deductive fashion to arrive at a summary of ten, shall we say *The Ten Commandments?* No. Too presumptuous, maybe just small letters, *the ten commandments.* Yes. Let's go with that. So, as did Moses come down the mountain with the Ten Commandments from God, carved into stone, so do I come before you with these commandments that may as well be from God, whether that be the God of Abraham, or the God of Mother Earth, or the No God of primordial soup and evolution, because we were either made by God to work this way, or evolved from the primordial soup of nothingness to work *just this way.* It is all so beautiful, utterly and magnificently so.

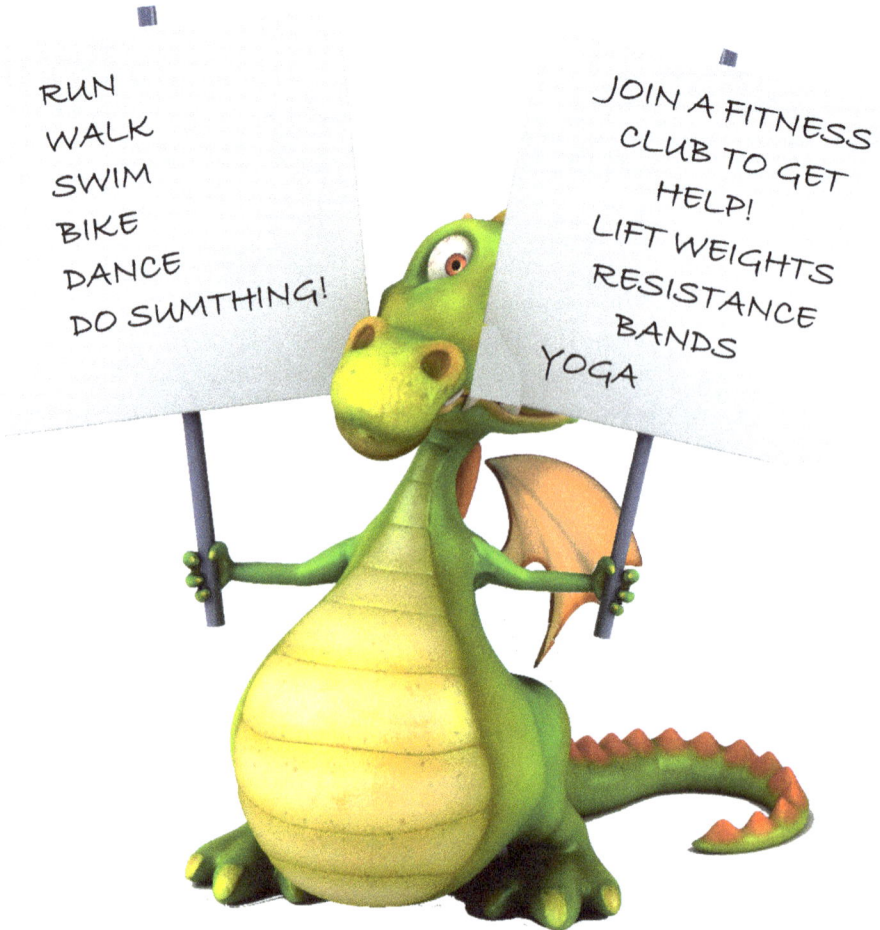

RUN
WALK
SWIM
BIKE
DANCE
DO SUMTHING!

JOIN A FITNESS CLUB TO GET HELP!
LIFT WEIGHTS
RESISTANCE BANDS
YOGA

The ten commandments

1. PICK A DIET PLAN: MY BIAS IS TOWARDS A LOW-CARB KETOGENIC, ANTI-INFLAMMATORY STRATEGY. IT IS MY FEELING THAT THESE DIETS ARE EASIER TO COMPLY WITH AS THEY ARE LESS RESTRICTIVE THAN THE PLANT-BASED, ANIMAL-PRODUCT-AVOIDANCE STRATEGY; BUT, YOU'RE THE BOSS. PICK WHATEVER YOU WANT.

2. PREPARE YOUR CASTLE: MAKE YOUR HOME A SAFE PLACE. IT IS YOUR FORTRESS OF SOLITUDE THAT SHOULD BE IMPERVIOUS TO THE DRAGON. HAVE A STRATEGY FOR HOW YOU'RE GOING TO EAT WHEN OUTSIDE THE WALL.

3. USE AN ON-LINE BASAL CALORIC NEED CALCULATOR TO FIGURE OUT HOW MANY CALORIES YOU SHOULD CONSUME PER DAY TO LOSE 1-2 POUNDS PER WEEK: IF YOU ARE ON ONE OF THE DIETS TOWARDS EITHER EXTREME OF LOW-FAT, PLANT-BASED; OR, LOW-CARB KETOGENIC, COUNTING CALORIES IS LESS IMPORTANT, BUT I THINK IT IS STILL HELPFUL FOR A FEW WEEKS, UNTIL YOU HAVE AN APPRECIATION OF HOW MANY CALORIES ARE IN THE FOODS YOU EAT. <HTTPS://WWW.NIDDK.NIH.GOV/BWP>

4. BE HONEST. BE TRUE TO YOURSELF. CONTROL WHAT YOU EAT.

5. UNDERSTAND THE EFFECT INSULIN HAS ON YOUR FAT METABOLISM: IT'S BAD. INSULIN MAKES FAT.

6. LIMIT YOUR CARBOHYDRATES TO LESS THAN 100 GRAMS/DAY: ZERO SUGAR OR REFINED CARBOHYDRATES.

7. IMPLEMENT AN INTERMITTENT FASTING STRATEGY: ALTERNATING DAYS OF FASTING, OR A DAILY 16-18 HOUR EXTENDED NIGHTTIME FAST.

8. UNDERSTAND THAT THE DRAGON OF OBESITY WILL KILL YOU: YOU WILL LIVE LESS, AND YOU WILL LIVE LESS WELL THAN YOU OTHERWISE WOULD.

9. EXERCISE IS GOOD AND NECESSARY, BUT IT'S NOT AS IMPORTANT AS YOUR DIET. *DO SOMETHING.*

10. RESISTANCE TRAINING PRESERVES LEAN MUSCLE MASS: IMPLEMENT A RESISTANCE TRAINING PROGRAM SO YOU DON'T TURN INTO A DORSAL-KYPHOTIC QUASIMODO.

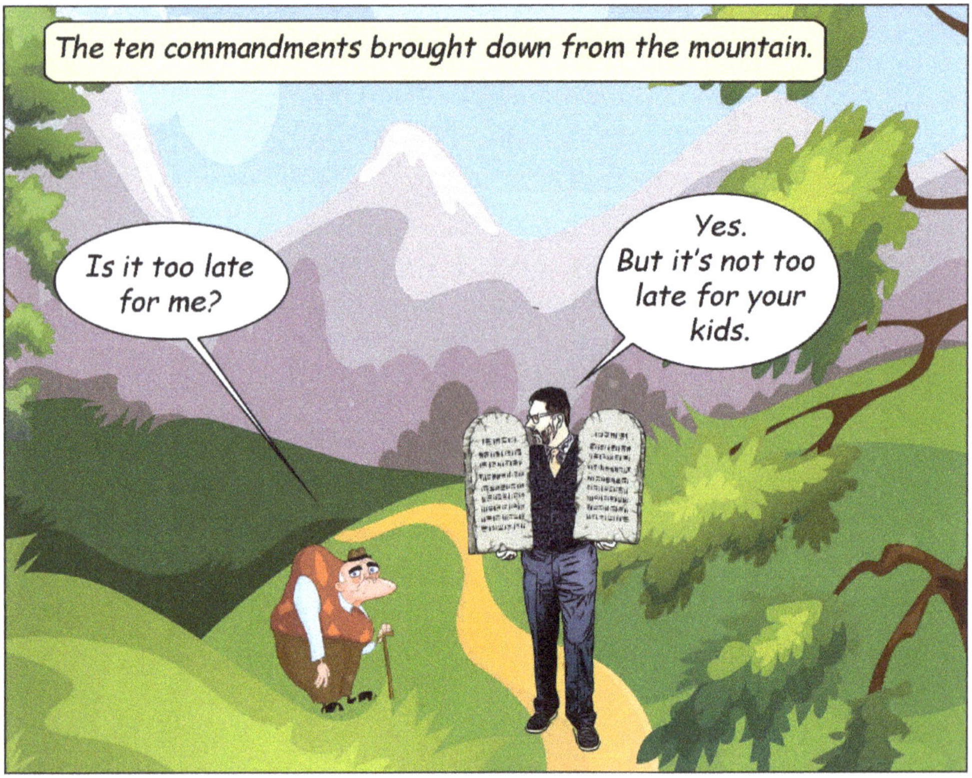
The ten commandments brought down from the mountain.
Is it too late for me?
Yes. But it's not too late for your kids.

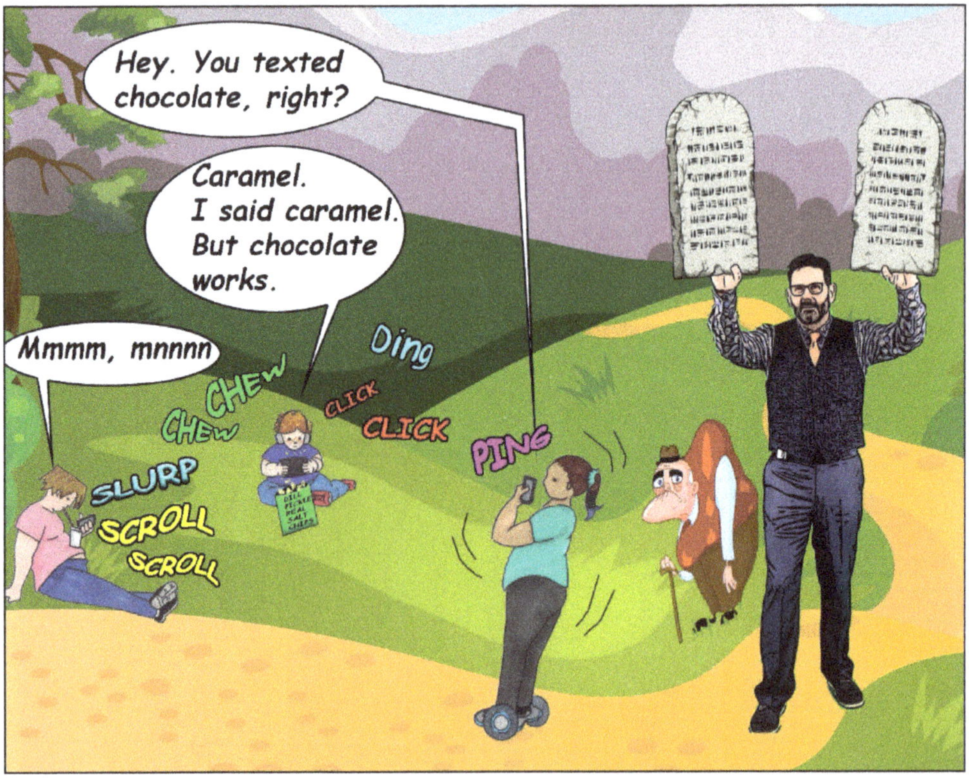
Hey. You texted chocolate, right?
Caramel. I said caramel. But chocolate works.
Mmmm, mnnnn
Ding
CHEW
CHEW
CLICK
CLICK
PING
SLURP
SCROLL
SCROLL

There you have it. The arrow of truth, in as few words as I could make it. If you are obese, especially if morbidly so, you will more likely die from an obesity-related illness or cancer than you otherwise would. If you are obese, especially if morbidly so, you will live less well, and less long than you otherwise would. If you are obese, especially if morbidly so, it doesn't have to be that way. You can change. You can change your thoughts, and with that you will change your world, and live longer and live better than you otherwise would.

This arrow alone should be enough to slay your dragon. It was for me. I never looked back. I drove that arrow deep into the beating heart of my dragon, killing it dead, feeling the pulsing ebb of its life leaving. If you think the arrow of truth is enough for you, you may stop reading.

However, there will be times when you might be weak, vulnerable, prone to the various baits and temptations of the dragon, which leads us to the second arrow. This is the fun one, for me at least. I always liked the stuff that is the substance of the arrow of reality.

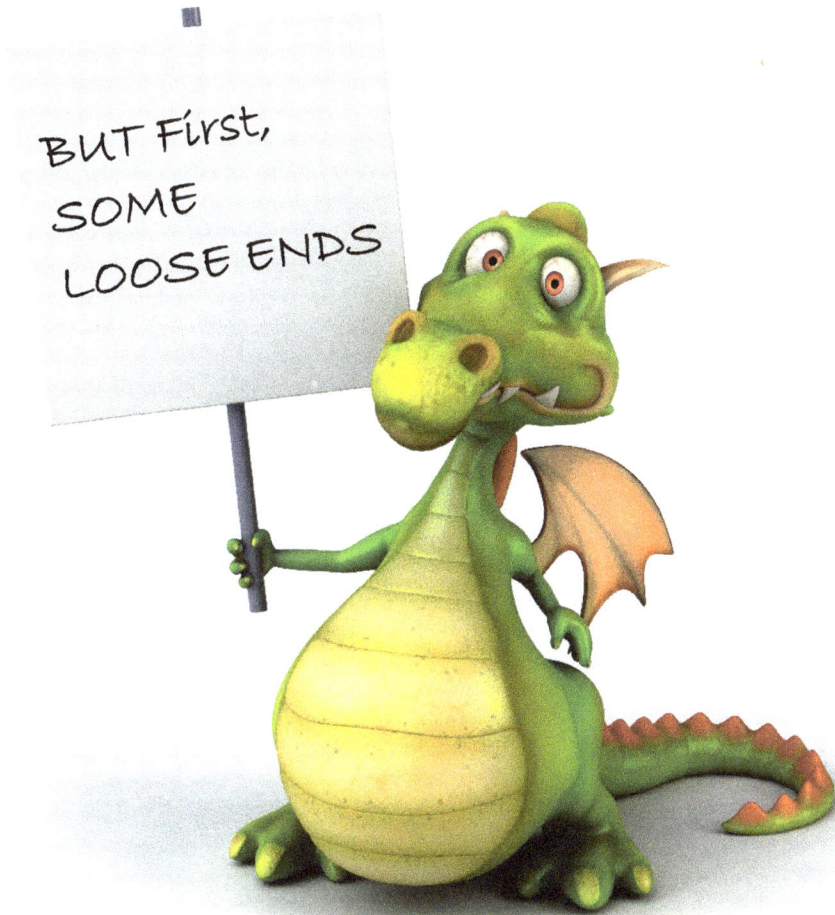

BUT First, SOME LOOSE ENDS

What exactly is mindfulness, and what am I supposed to do with that?

The definition of *mindfulness* is a state of mind that is achieved by being aware of the present moment, acknowledging one's feelings, thoughts and bodily sensations. A mindful diet is being aware of the stress and unhappiness and belief systems such that you might apply strategies and manage your behavior relative to your diet in a positive fashion. This is something that we will be addressing more completely later. Believe me. However, I introduce it here from the standpoint of stress reduction, and the vital roles that sleep and exercise play in that. It is important that you not deprive yourself of sleep, and I mean more than logging six to eight hours (closer to eight) in the horizontal position, which is to say the *quality* of your sleep. If you are overweight or obese, you are high-risk for the comorbidity of Obstructive Sleep Apnea (OSA). If you are not already being treated for OSA and if you are chronically fatigued or are told that you snore, then ask your primary care provider to evaluate you for OSA.

The value of exercise is more than that of energy expenditure. There is also value in the enjoyment and sense of well-being and accomplishment that is achieved with regular exercise. It is well established in the medical literature that exercise exerts physiologic effects on the central nervous system that positively impact anxiety and depression, as little as two to two-and-a-half hours a week (11). Two-and-a-half hours a week is not a lot, as I implied earlier in *Phase IV*. Again, it is important that you *do something*, aerobic and resistance training both.

Both sleep and exercise are not to be underestimated and are of vital importance to the attainment of your goals.

> Both EXERCISE and SLEEP are important factors for an overall sense of wellbeing and stress reduction, which are integral to any sort of mindfulness. We must learn *to be still*.

How is this going to work for my family?

The most important thing is that, ultimately, mindful, healthy eating is the goal. Why should this be different for your family? There is no reason why your family shouldn't eat well too, especially the children; however, let's talk practicality.

Kids will be kids, and spouses will be spouses. If your spouse is obese or overweight, they should be doing what you are doing, and if they do not, that is no reason why you still can't be successful. I think that intermittent fasting is the answer because it removes all meals from the equation but one, maybe two. All you must ask of your family is to eat one healthy meal a day, with you, and that most likely would be dinner. Skipping breakfast with a coffee and creamer/coconut oil additive and water w/fiber is easy enough. You usually aren't that hungry in the morning anyway. The children and the spouse can have a high-fiber cereal in which case it shouldn't be your daily task. It should be the eating spouse and/or the child's. If the spouse is *in it* with you, then you can whip something up for the kids, if a healthy cold cereal doesn't work. It may be that your child is old enough to be on autopilot already, so breakfast isn't a problem.

Usually, lunch is not an issue because the kids are in school and both you and your spouse are at work, or one or the other is; therefore, you have the option of a sensible lunch on your own, or simply fasting through lunch too, which is more aggressive and something I'm not doing currently.

A strategy of INTERMITTENT FASTING can be used by a *dieting-member* of a *non-dieting* family as it distills the day down to ONE important meal. It is the least your family can do for you.

The only meal that counts is dinner with the family, and since you've logged an 18 hour fast, or thereabouts, you can cut loose a little because this is the time you will have insulin, so it doesn't matter so much if you have a diet soda, or a starchy vegetable like a sweet potato or wild rice or grain or modest serving of whole wheat pasta or bread. Have a donut *(I'm kidding, kind of)*. This is the time to do it. This is your time with the family. You can prepare a meal such as this very easily and quickly with a little forethought. It's easier if your spouse/significant other participates.

I've thought about this a lot. *How can an entire family go on a diet?* This is a good answer, intermittent fasting, because it compresses two to three meals down to one. Snacking is discouraged. You will have two meals a day, at most. It will be more manageable. The kids can eat what they will, but you won't be part of it other than the delivery process. Besides, the kids need to learn how to eat well from early on, because if they don't, they could be screwed up for years.

The hardest part of intermittent fasting will probably be the evening after dinner: popcorn at the movies, milk and cookies before bed, a quick trip to the DQ, etc. The evening is the hardest for me, and my wife and I are empty nesters, so I know it will be more difficult with a larger family; but, if you have a reasonable, full dinner meal, it will be easier. It will become a question of your drive, motivation and desire, and of course, there remains the last two arrows in your quiver.

Maybe I should do one of those really low-calorie diets to get started and lose a lot of weight right off the bat.

You mean a Very Low-Calorie Diet (**VLCD**) that typically involves the heavy use of a straw and oral suction and flavors like strawberry and vanilla. Yummy, sign me up. **Not!** Seriously, these diets are less than 1000 Calories/day and typically consist of a combination of shakes and packaged meals of foods that definitely don't look like they came from the ground or were recently killed, but they are low calorie and have protein, fewer carbs and are likely low-fat.

The problem with a VLCD is that your hypothalamus will interpret the severe caloric restriction as starvation/famine and will decrease your basal metabolic rate (BMR), resetting it lower. This effect is fairly immediate, a matter of days, but the reverse is not the case. When you start eating more, your metabolic rate does not automatically increase like it decreased initially. This effect is called *adaptive thermogenesis*, and I discuss it more fully at *FatThief.com*.

A VLCD or a severe caloric restriction beyond a few days will reset your Basal Metabolic Rate lower and losing weight will be even harder. When you stop, you quickly regain any weight lost, and more. *Don't do it.*

Fasting, with a mild caloric restriction, does not cause this response because you eat a more appropriate amount at some time during the day. If you simply follow your diet strategy, and implement an intermittent fasting program, you will increase your body's tendency to metabolize fat over time because of the decreased insulin exposure. It is the frequent feeding of regular diets, and the VLCDs--because you're so damn hungry all the time that you have to eat something every few hours, like a dog getting a treat—which allows for a continuous level of insulin and therefore a continuous suppression of fat metabolism. Of course, this is combined with a recently lowered basal metabolic rate, so you lose even less, and when you stop the artificial feedings...WATCH OUT. You'll re-inflate like a balloon from the compressed air cylinder next to the funnel-cake fryer at the carnival before you can say, "Mississippi;" or nearly so, it seems.

The only case where the BMR wouldn't drop as much on a VLCD is if it is a **K**etogenic VLCD (**VLCDK**) I did find a study performed on less than 20 participants that demonstrated only a mild decrease in the BMR (12). It is thought that this was secondary to a relative preservation of the lean muscle mass which a ketogenic diet engenders, in contrast to a non-ketogenic VLCD.

In summary, VLCDs: I wouldn't recommend them. I don't see the reason or benefit of unnatural eating at a higher cost.

I sure am glad God invented diet soda; couldn't get by without it.

Ummm…you're gonna have to, at least most of the time. It is quite conclusive; many studies have demonstrated that diet soda is no better than regular soda (13). As little as one can a day is still associated with similar rates of the metabolic syndrome, and there is no benefit relative to weight-loss as compared with regular soda. It is thought that the sweetness may be stimulatory for appetite and even the artificial sweeteners may cause the release of insulin.

If you still want one, have it within the window of your breaking of the fast when elevated insulin levels are already present.

I used to be a huge diet soda fan. I still miss it. I still have one every other day or so, with a meal. What I have done instead is significantly increased my water intake because there's not much else, other than coffee and tea; however, I have found that putting a large pitcher of fruit-infused water in the fridge does make it more exciting and slightly special. I prefer lemons, two quarters, in the water, changed daily.

> Even diet soda has been shown to be associated with the metabolic syndrome, as little as one can per day.

Is beating the dragon going to be expensive?

The fact that I am asking should be your first clue. I'm only asking because I wanted to be able to tell you most emphatically, *IT IS NOT.*

Oftentimes, unhealthy choices seem cheaper than the healthy ones, but you are eating smaller portions and you are eating less frequently.

In fact, I would venture to say that it will be less expensive than whatever you currently are doing. That is what I have found.

Think about it: you don't eat breakfast, you don't need that ridiculous box of snacks filled with 100 calorie carbohydrate bars or 250 calorie meal replacement bars at $1.50 each, no bakery goods, chips, cookies, etc. You'll have lunch and one meal a day that counts--chicken, fish, salmon, grass-fed beef, bison, lean ground beef, eggs, dairy; a side of vegetables or similar, a starchy something or other like squash or sweet potato, some fruit for a dessert, and maybe once or twice a week some type of a ketogenic dessert, if necessary.

Eating as I've described, without snacking, normal sized portions, and implementing a fasting strategy is not expensive.

An added benefit of a fasting strategy is *time*. Less time preparing meals equals more productivity in your life.

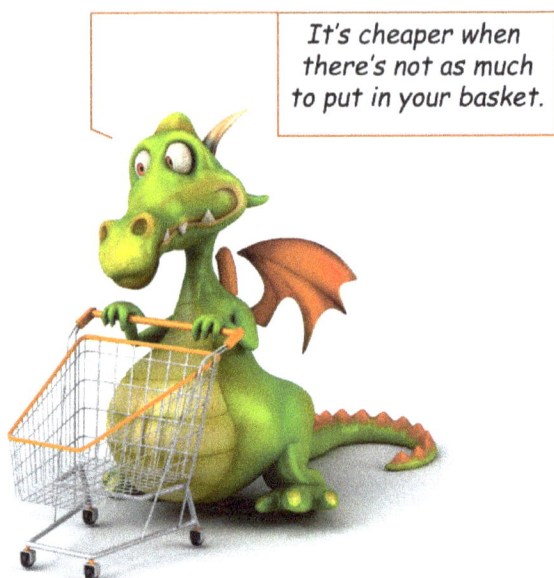

It's cheaper when there's not as much to put in your basket.

What if it's a gland problem?

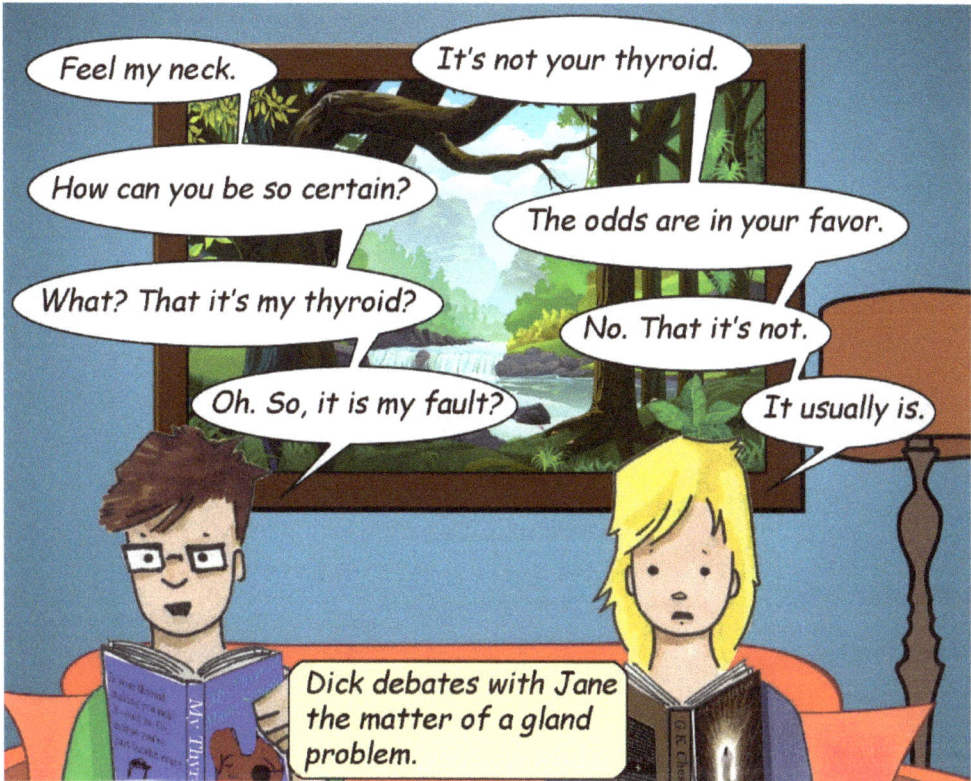

Feel my neck.

It's not your thyroid.

How can you be so certain?

The odds are in your favor.

What? That it's my thyroid?

No. That it's not.

Oh. So, it is my fault?

It usually is.

Dick debates with Jane the matter of a gland problem.

Ahhh…you must mean your thyroid. That's the obvious one; unfortunately, there is, at the most, only a modest effect of treatment with thyroid hormone in inducing weight-loss in *overt hypothyroidism* and no established benefit in subclinical hypothyroidism. In fact, there is some thought that obesity may be a cause of hypothyroidism rather than hypothyroidism being a cause of it (14).

There is a natural human tendency perhaps to assign blame to something other than ourselves. If you really think it might be a gland problem, such as the thyroid, or the much more uncommon case of a tumor of the pituitary gland, which can cause an excess production of steroid hormones (Cushing Syndrome) causing obesity; then ask your primary care provider to test your for those things, if appropriate.

A more pertinent question, relative to blame, would be: *Is it in my DNA?* and the answer to that is *it could be.*

There are very rare genetic syndromes associated with severe obesity; however, they typically present in childhood, so if you weren't morbidly obese as a three-year-old, you don't have this.

What is more common is a variable genetic disposition to obesity (15). Some people gain weight easier than others. This is kind of like the *luck of the draw* and until there is a way to reverse engineer your DNA, you must play the hand you're dealt. It follows that losing weight will be harder for some than it is for others; however, I would only ask you to Google *"pictures of people from 1950."*

Here, let me do it for you. Tell me, please, how many obese people do you see?

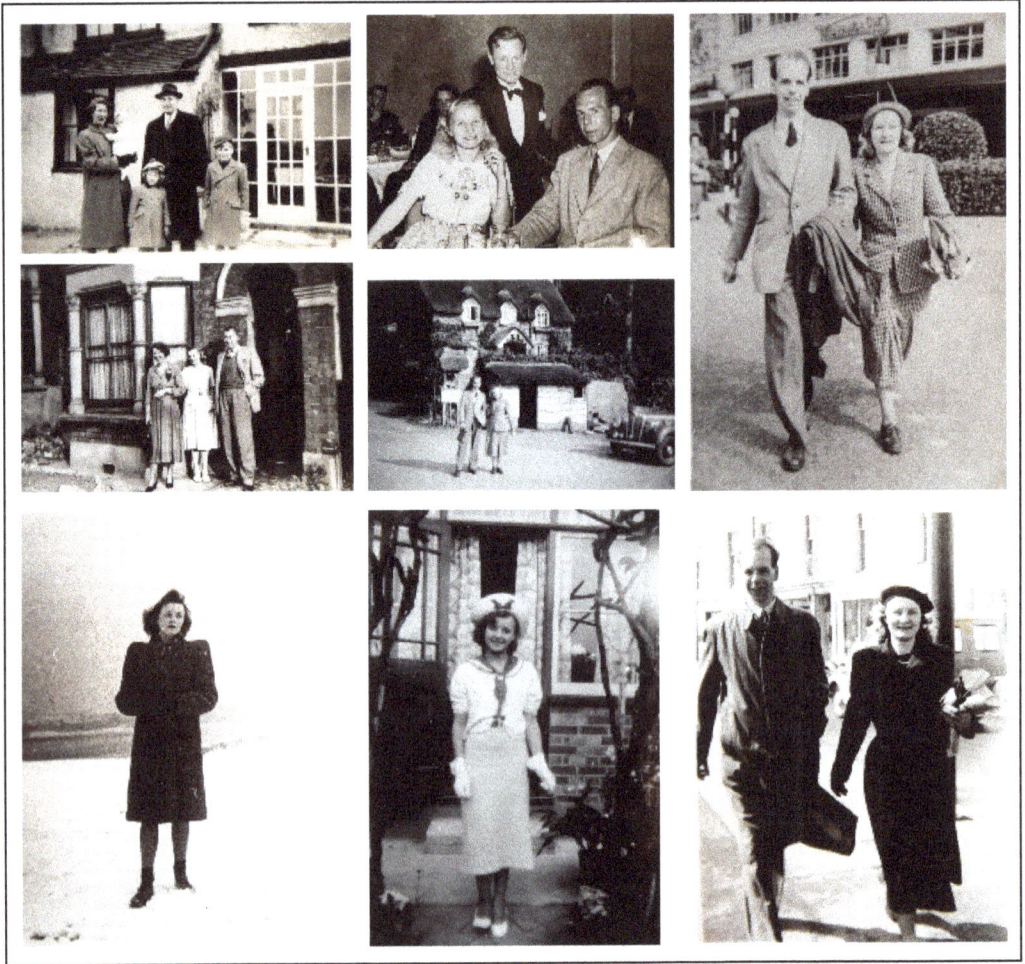

Ah-Haa. Given that evolution is measured in multiples of millennia, if genetics is a factor there should be just as many obese people in 1950 as there are in 2019, a span of a mere 69 years. What your lying eyes are telling you is that obesity is, for the most part, environmental.

Should I take an Over The Counter (OTC) dietary supplement to help me lose weight?

No.

Seriously. No. There may be a role at some point for a physician-supervised pharmacological intervention; however, few Over The Counter (**OTC**) dietary supplements demonstrate clinical efficacy unless they increase the metabolic rate, such as ephedrine (not good), caffeine, and green tea extract. A few others may demonstrate some marginal effect *as long as you are taking them*, but only marginal. Save your money, eat healthy, eat well, live well, think well; that is how you beat your dragon.

> OTC dietary supplements are not regulated and of questionable efficacy in most cases. I do not recommend any and do not sell any. Just say NO.

Maybe I should just have an operation?

There's a reason I ask this question last, in fact, these first 90-some pages have been in a very specific order and the reason this is last is because it should be last. It should be the last thing you would do because if you can do all these things I have described, it is far more likely that you will not need an operation than it is that you do. Bariatric surgery is not magical, it is mainly mechanical. It still requires a diet after; so, why not diet first and see if that works?

Not everyone needs to be on a ketogenic diet. Not everyone needs to employ an intermittent fasting strategy. Some people will do both those things and then back off to a sensible, mindful way of eating after attaining a goal. There is a different solution for different people. As the King said to the White Rabbit in Alice in Wonderland, all you need to do is "Begin at the beginning, and go on till you come to the end: then stop." In our case, *STOP* means the cessation of a caloric restriction, but a *continuation* of our new, mindful way of thinking.

Bariatric surgery refers to an operation for obesity.

Bariatric surgery should be the last thing you consider. If you do the things I've described, it is more likely that an operation will not be required. What is required *is resolve, conviction, and a healthy self-worth*.

If you start at the beginning, you should find success with advancement through the phases. It may be that a non-ketogenic, caloric-responsible, no bad fats, refined sugars, etc. works for you. It may be that you have to step up to a low-carb diet, and that will work for you. It may be that you have to step that up to a limited fast, as simple as not eating after dinner, and that will work for you. It may be that you require an extended, 18 hour fast or a more strict ketogenic diet to meet your objectives, and that will work for you.

Lastly, it really may be that all this doesn't work for you. This would be EXTREMELY unlikely. It may be that the genetic burden you bear for obesity is too much to overcome, and there indeed may be a role for a surgical intervention; however, this is much less the case than is currently reflected in the gross volumes of bariatric surgery being performed today, in my estimation. I do not feel that many of the hundreds of thousands of patients having a bariatric procedure (over 200,000 annually) have an insurmountable genetic burden, or that diets *don't work for them*. I think that they aren't dieting the right way, and the evidence in that, in my view, is the significant rate of recidivism (relapse rate) of obesity *after* surgery, which suggests to me that it is, after all, the diet, in many cases.

It is done. You now hold the arrow of truth in your hands. It is yours. You know what to do. You know how to do it. And, most importantly, you know *why* to do it. It is so doable that there is no reason to not do it. Pick up your arrow. It is time to battle your dragon.

Pull out your phone and watch the 1st video at FatThief.com

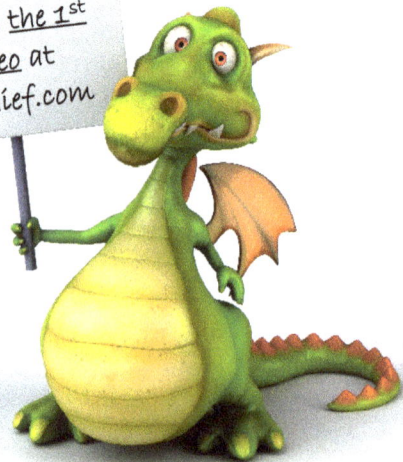

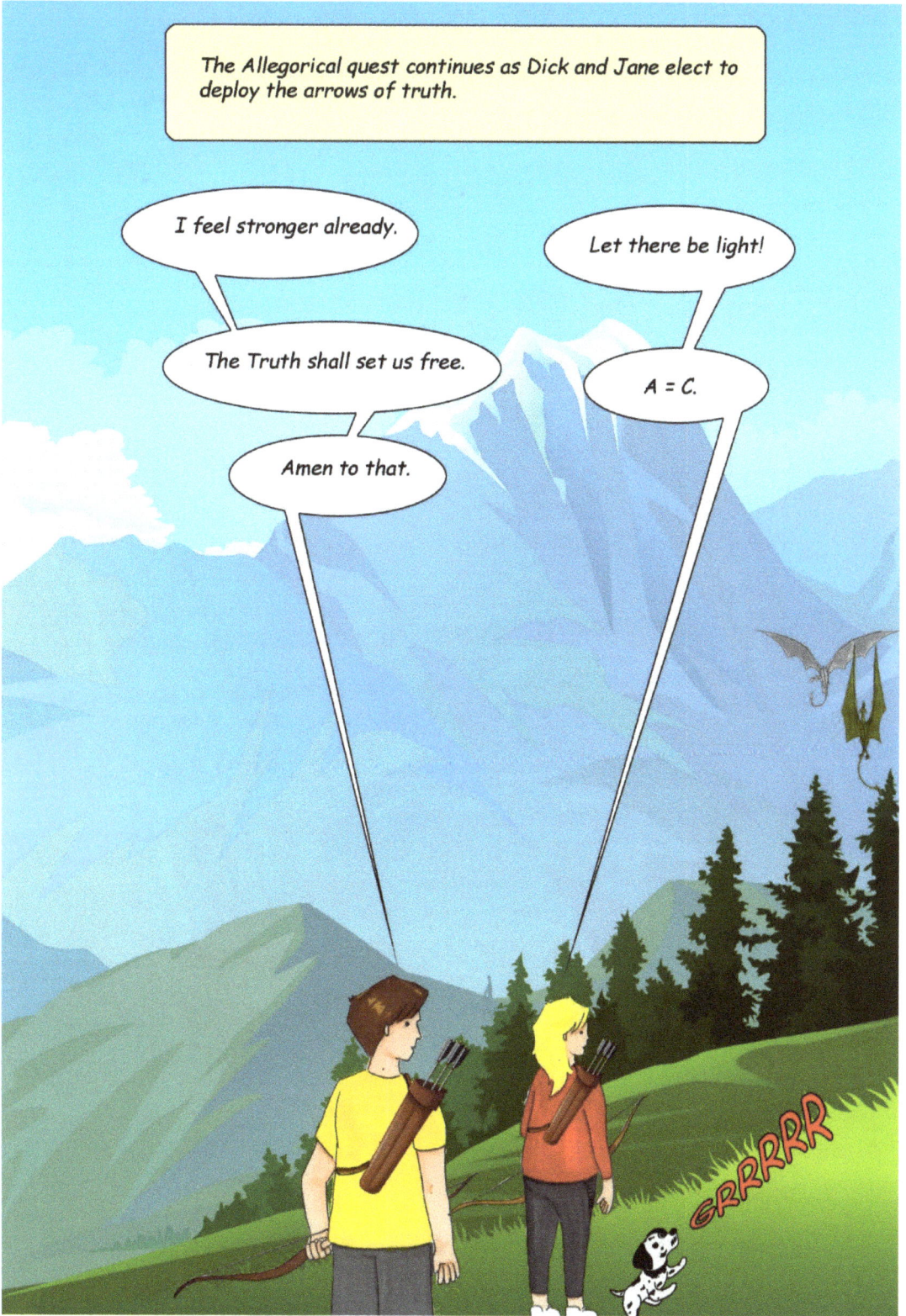

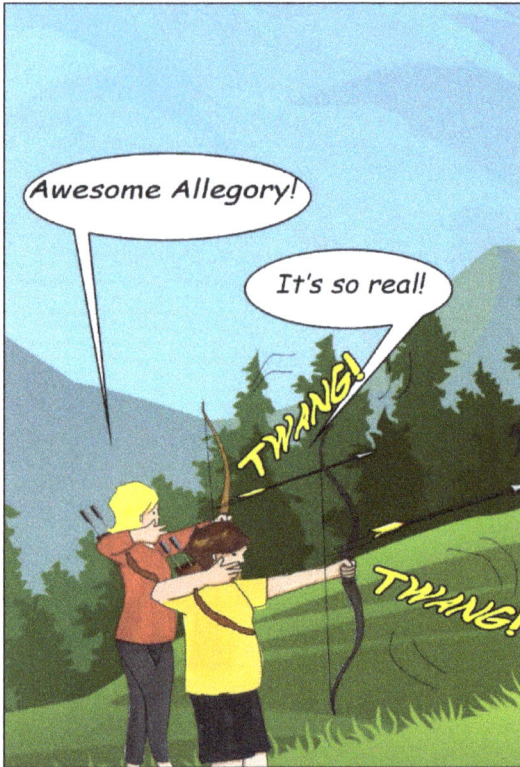

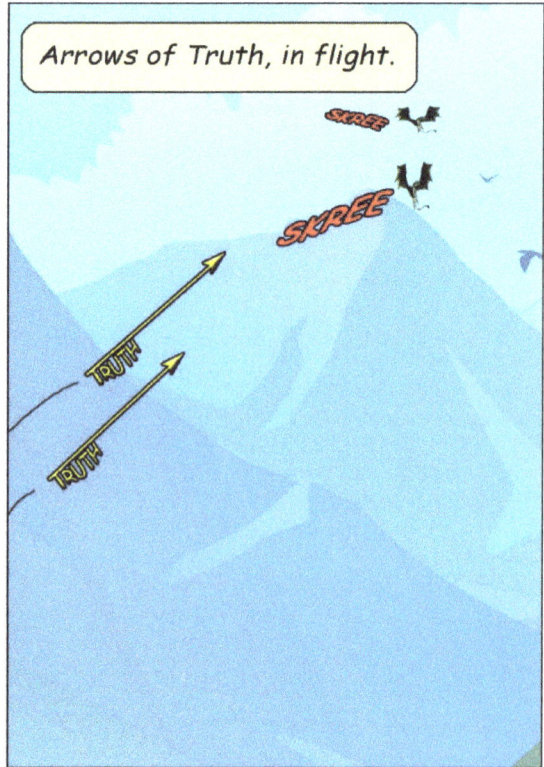

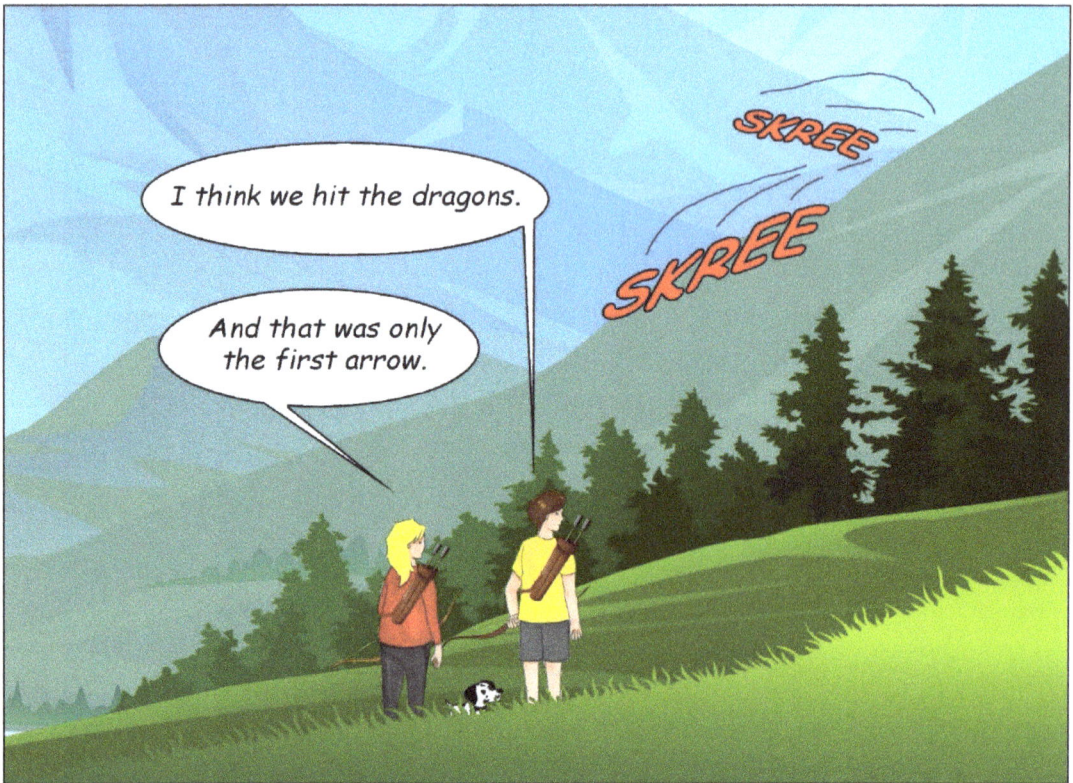

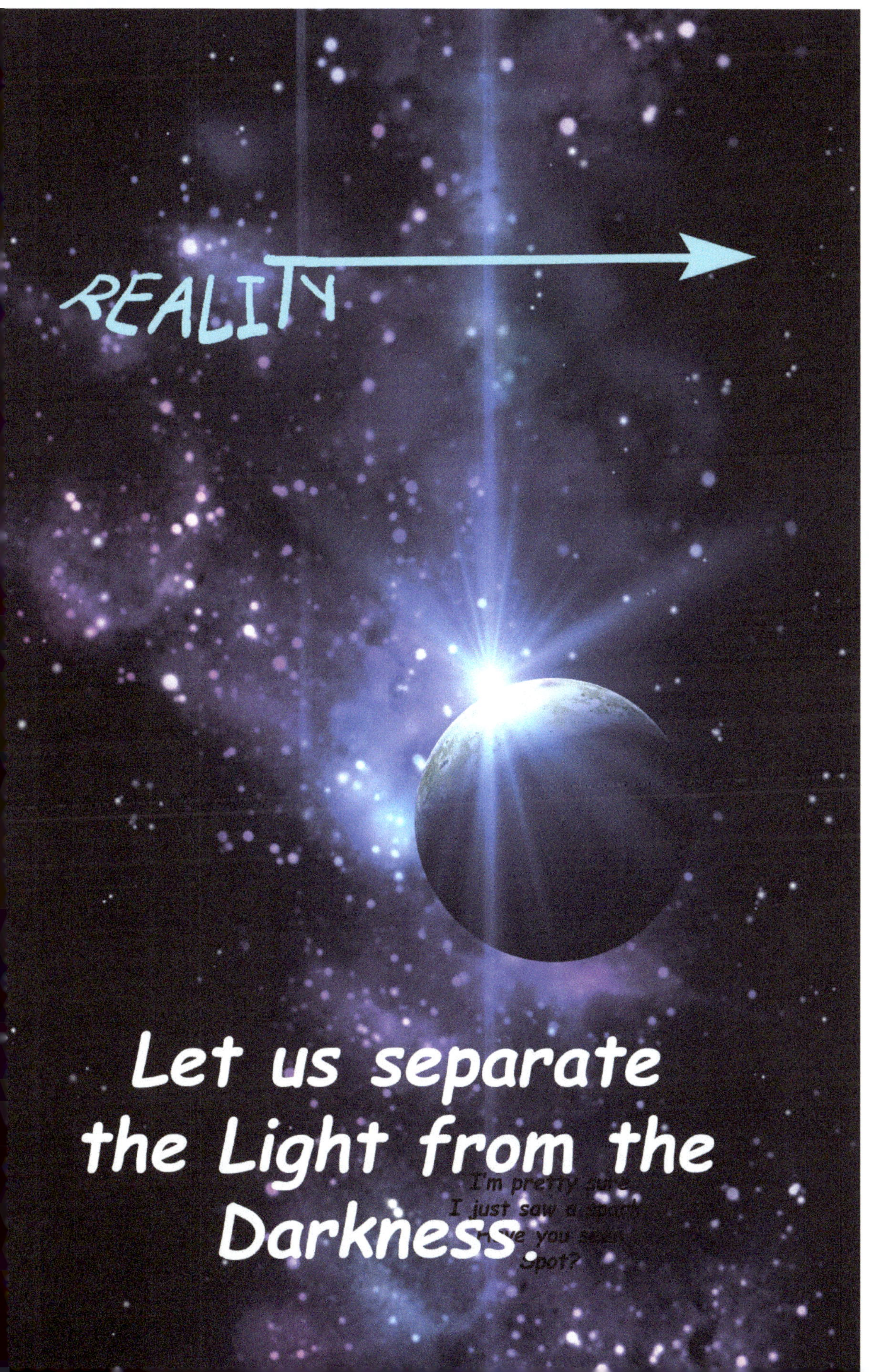
REALITY
Let us separate the Light from the Darkness.
I'm pretty sure
I just saw a
you
Spot?

CHAPTER SEVEN: SELF-SELECTION OF REALITY

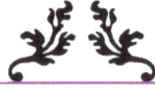

Vice is a monster of so frightful mien,
As, to be hated, needs but to be seen;
Yet seen too oft, familiar with her face,
We first endure, then pity, then embrace.

Alexander Pope, Essay on Man, Epistle II

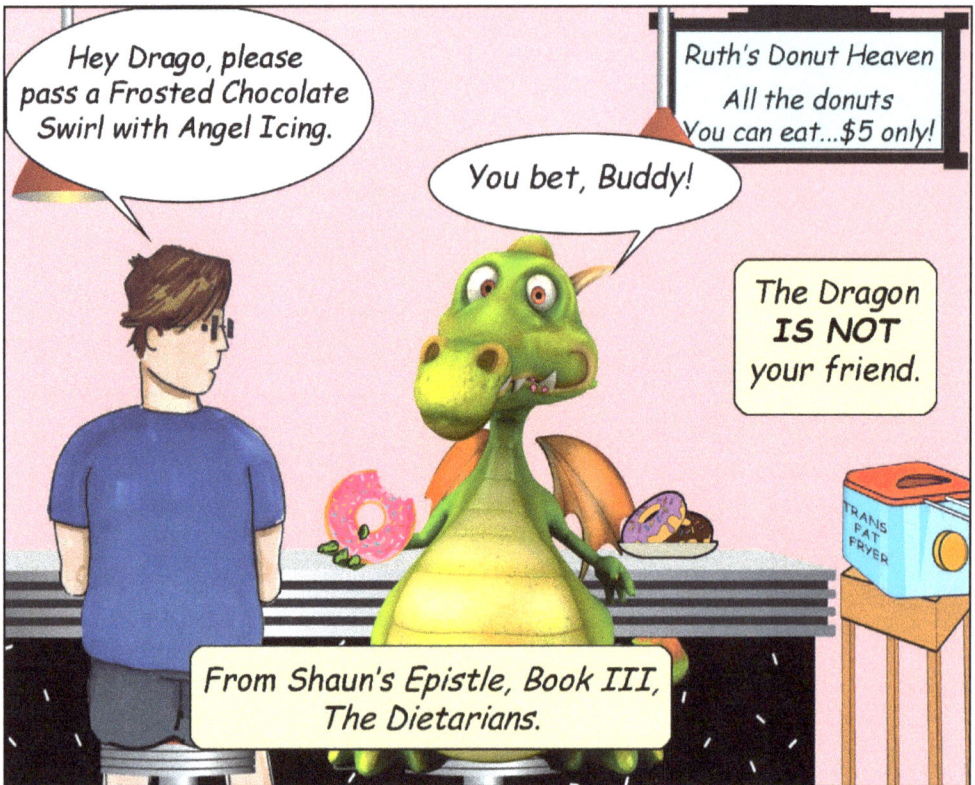

We all have a little *crazy* in us, and I can only say that because I've got a little crazy myself, and I used to have a lot more. The important thing is that you must recognize the possibility of that and if it is detrimental to your health and life in general. What I'm trying to say is that you must know thyself. This is the primary focus of the balance of my epistle to you, kind of like one of St. Paul's letters, not because I'm a saint, but because I care very much. I could even call this section, Shaun's *Letter to the Dietarians, Book III*, with the purpose of knowing thyself because it is by increasing your fund of self-knowledge that you will be better able to heal thyself.

It is my fervent wish that your own personal dragon of obesity is simply the result of a deficit of knowledge, a dragon easily dispatched with the arrow of truth, but what if it's not. *What if it's more than that?*

Is there an emotional element—sadness, anger, hopelessness--that plays a role? What if you experience repetitive negative thinking or have bad automatic thoughts running through your mind? What if you need more help than some few pages can deliver?

> IF YOU SUFFER FROM SEVERE DEPRESSION OR LOW SELF-WORTH OR SUICIDAL IDEATION, PLEASE SEE YOUR DOCTOR FOR PERSONALIZED PROFESSIONAL ATTENTION.

Further self-study may be required, even professional help with a Behavioral Therapist or Psychologist. You can access these specialists through your primary care provider, and it should be covered by most health insurance policies, subject to deductibles of course. This is easy if you've had a baby, or a hernia repair, or a colonoscopy within the deductible year because that means that your deductible is likely maxed out, so I'd go all in. I'd have all those moles you've been watching for a few years removed. I'd schedule a cardiac ablation (at least 60k) for chronic atrial fibrillation, maybe a knee replacement, or two, or how about a surgical intervention for reflux disease? Just go out and get it all done. Unfortunately, that's the current state of the high-deductible plans; the insured are incentivized to do nothing other than preventive health measures; or, to do everything.

But I digress, we must return to reality and what I want to share with you about the reality you inhabit. In this manual, I am suggesting to you the presence of a gateway to multiple realities, all available to you, realities dependent on the choices you make.

I would like to now shift your considerable focus, like a laser beam, to this gateway of multiple realities stretching before you at this exact moment in time because with the next turn of the page a new reality is created. You'll see what I mean.

> **Metaphysical**, another word for philosophical; relating to the fundamental origin of things and reality and existence and free will; kind of like *the meaning of life*.

We inhabit a reality that is largely a product of the choices we make. I would like to offer a metaphysical argument of this statement because I think it is a fascinating discussion, and quite cool.

There occurs a daily battle that rages within us; multiple skirmishes against multiple fronts, some major assaults, some minor, losses and wins, triumphs and tragedies. It is the choices we make that determine the outcomes of each individual conflict. It is the outcome of the daily battle in its entirety that determines the course of our own reality on a day to day basis, which translates into longer term outcomes. The implication is that we have the capability to change our reality. It is this capability that represents the second arrow that you might place in your quiver for slaying dragons.

> This is so utterly fascinatingly super cool. Please relax, enjoy the pictures, and if you are as enchanted as I am, *Google it and read and explore* beyond these few pages.

Historically, there have been two dominant versions of reality (16), one definitely more dominant than the other, and more recently, perhaps a third version that is even more sci-fi than the less dominant historical version. Let me begin with the dominant version first, called the *Copenhagen Interpretation*, and we'll limit our discussion to a story about a cat who belonged to a man called Schrodinger.

I should say that it was an imaginary cat, because a bad thing happens to the cat half the time. This famous thought experiment was proposed in 1935 and all the genius minds, including Einstein's, argued over the implications.

Are you ready? This is so cool. I know I already said that, but I'm an emphatic sort of guy, if you haven't noticed.

Imagine a cat, any cat will do, but perhaps not your own cat lest that prove too painful. Imagine a steel box large enough to comfortably contain the cat and some accessory equipment, a closed system that you cannot see inside of with only one door that you open to put the cat inside and subsequently to remove the cat. For the cat, those four walls represent the limits of its universe. It is all that exists.

The accessory equipment includes a glass vial of poison above which is poised a hammer that is controlled by a relay switch that is activated by a minute portion of radioactive substance. The radioactive material is so small that there is only a 50% probability that an atom will decay in the course of an hour. If it does decay, a particle will be released that will trip the relay switch causing the hammer to fall, which breaks the glass vial, which releases the poison, which vaporizes. Bye-bye kitty.

Although there could be many variables, for the purposes of the thought experiment, the outcome is a binary outcome. It is either/or. Either the cat is alive when the door is opened after one hour and the result observed, or the cat is dead. Dr. Schrodinger maintained that while the cat was in the box, it existed in a state of superposition of being half-alive and half-dead, and the reality is only realized when the result is observed. Inside the box, before the result is observed, there exists a range of possibilities in which every outcome is possible, which in this binary case is a live cat or a dead cat.

DISCLAIMER
REMEMBER. IT'S A THOUGHT EXPERIMENT. IT IS ONLY IMAGINED. NO KITTY, *OR PUPPY* DIES.   WELL, MAYBE IN A PARALELL UNIVERSE, BUT NOT IN THIS ONE, THE ONE THAT MATTERS, *TO US*.

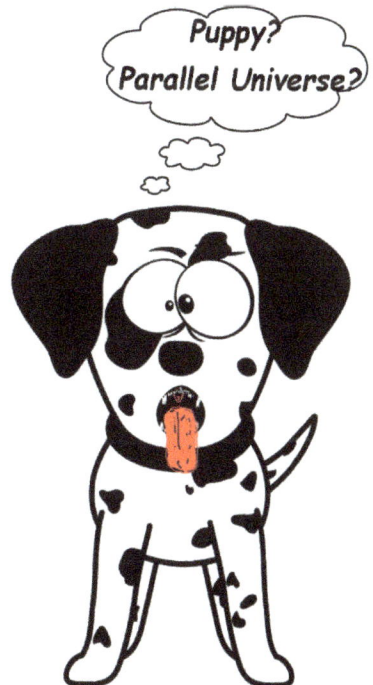

Puppy? Parallel Universe?

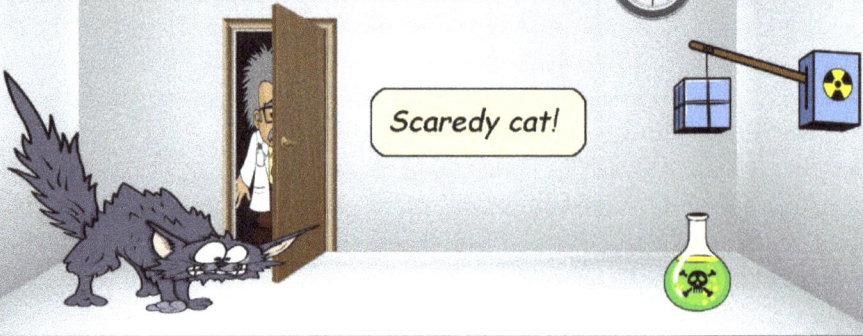

Version of Reality #1: Copenhagen Interpretation
A Reality of Probabilities

1. The cat is placed in the box.

Scaredy cat!

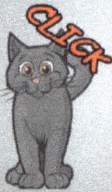

1/2 Alive and 1/2 Dead

2. At the moment the observer leaves the room, the cat exists in a state of super-position: 1/2 alive and half dead.

3. After 1 Hr. the result is observed: an exact 50% probability of either of two possible outcomes.

Every outcome is possible!

In this Binary case, only 2 outcomes are possible.

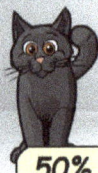

50% chance

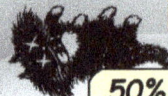

50% chance

> This **FIRST** version of reality, the **Copenhagen Interpretation**, is a reality of probabilities. *Anything* can happen, but what does happen is the *most probable,* based upon actions and choices made.

We do not live in a four-walled steel box universe of a binary outcome, of course. We exist in a limitless universe of limitless variables and outcomes, *ad infinitim.* What the Copenhagen Interpretation implies is that any result, any outcome, represents a range of probabilities of every possible outcome, and although anything is possible, it is simply that some outcomes are more likely than others. The reality of an inhabitant of the Copenhagen universe is a reality of probabilities. There is only one universe, and anything can happen, but whatever does happen is the most probable, most of the time. It's like shooting an arrow at a target. The most probable outcome is hitting the target, somewhere; however, there is a mathematical probability that the arrow could veer wildly off to the left or right, or even upwards through the atmosphere to spear the moon. It could happen, probabilistically.

The less dominant theory of reality is just as fun, if not even more so, and it was conceived of by Hugh Everett in 1957. This is the *Many Worlds Interpretation,* which is the stuff of science-fiction, as well as being a valid theory of our physical universe, or rather, our physical parallel univers(es).

> The **SECOND** version of reality, the **Many Worlds Interpretation**, is a reality of *multiple* (infinite) universes.
>
> *Every possible outcome* of an action or choice does happen, in some world/universe that you cannot see because *you exist in only one world/universe/reality.*

In contrast to the Copenhagen Interpretation in which the current reality is one of a range of possibilities, in the Many Worlds theory, the current reality is one of an infinite number of parallel worlds, parallel realities. In the binary (two) outcome reality of Schrodinger's cat, at the exact instant you open the door and a relieved live cat slinks out, a bifurcation occurs in which an alternate universe splits off in which you open the door to a faint whiff of something bad and find, sadly, a dead cat; but the first you is completely unaware of the second you.

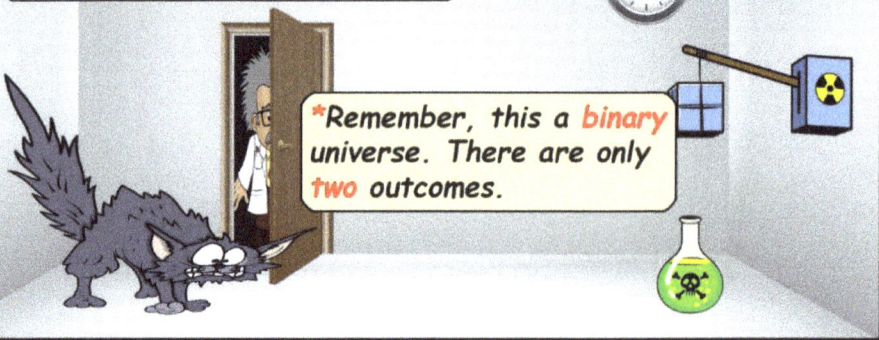

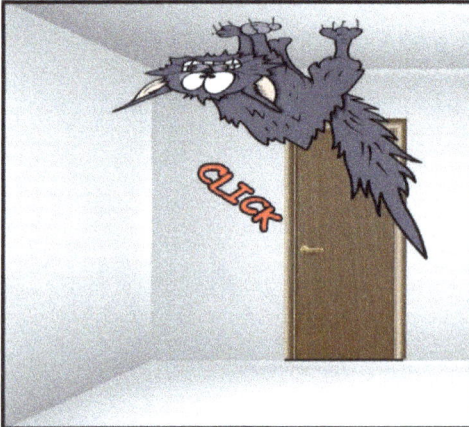

2. Cat is still scared because it doesn't know which **Reality** will be realilzed until the observer **chooses** to open the door..

3. At the exact moment the observer opens the door, the current reality bifurcates into a paralell reality of the other possible outcome..

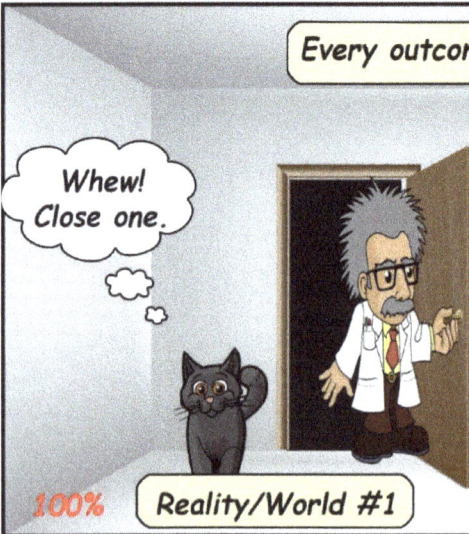

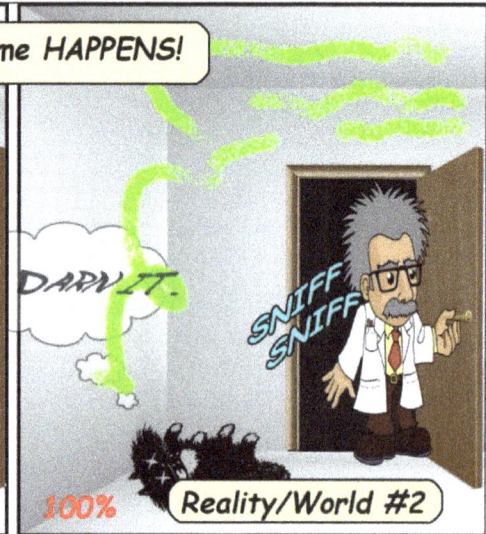

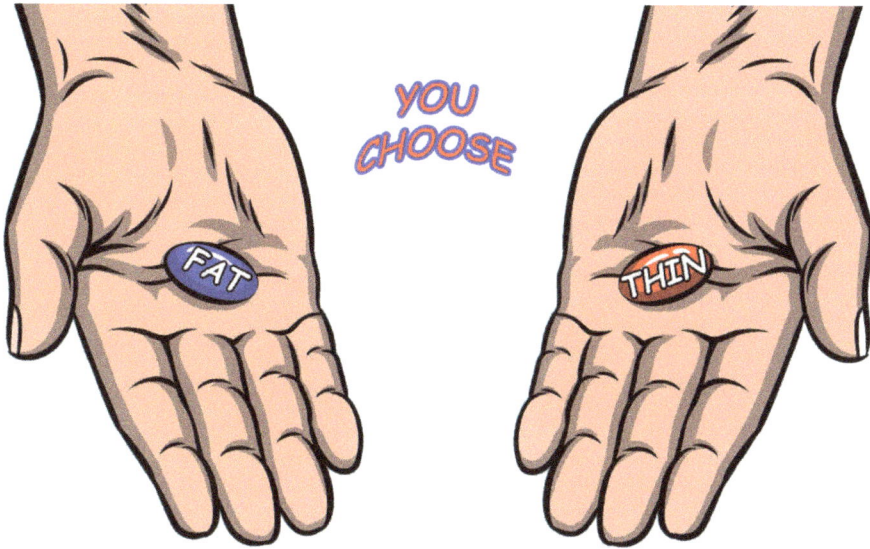

There are other interpretations of reality, all of them difficult to conceive of, including a theory that we are all living in a digital construct, not dissimilar to the cult-classic, *The Matrix*, starring Keanu Reeves as Neo who picks the Red pill (truth) over the Blue pill (fantasy).

So, you're sitting there or lying there and wondering *what arrow? What the hell are you talking about?* Well, besides the fact that I think it's fascinating, way more than I could allude to in a few paragraphs, the reality, as conceived of and proposed by geniuses of yesteryear and today, is either a reality of probabilities; or, a reality of multiple parallel universes, and the truth is that the latter theory is easier to reconcile mathematically.

The second arrow of Reality is the hard-metal tip that is **Free Will** and the power of choice. Consider the Copenhagen Interpretation--it's kind of like you are the cat, and the box is your brain. No one can see inside the box, all the observer sees is the cat, which is the manifestation of what goes on inside of the box (your brain and the choices you make). The outcome of what is observed is represented by a mathematical equation that represents a full range of probabilities or possible outcomes from the choices the brain makes, which are reflected in the cat (your external physical manifestation) that is visible to the observers.

So, if you make the decision to get that large bucket of popcorn, the one you can refill along with the regular Coke, after the previews *before* the movie actually starts and then go home that night and make the decision to have a dish of vanilla ice cream with Hershey's chocolate syrup and whipped cream with a cherry on top because all the carbs in the popcorn spiked your insulin and now you're hungry again; and then, in the morning…well, I'm sure you get my drift.

The point is, your reality is a product of the choices you make, choices made inside the box (your brain) that no one can see inside of; but, as observers of the universe, they do see the result, in this case, not a live cat or dead cat; rather, a fatter one or a thinner one. It is by making the right choices that you increase the probability of the desired outcome, thereby self-selecting the reality you want for yourself.

Alternatively, in a similar way, in the Many-worlds interpretation, the universe you inhabit is also a direct result of the choices you make; however, instead of exerting control by increasing the probability of a desired outcome by making the right choices, you make the proper choice *(most of the time)* and your reality continually branches, ad-infinitum, until you get to a desired reality. Like where a couple of guys stop you on the street and the taller one says, "Hi, we're the Russo brothers, and we're wondering if you'd like to star as a superhero in our new *Avengers* movie." Meanwhile, several branches removed, in a parallel reality on the multi-verse tree, far distant, is an alternate you who made all the wrong choices, struggling to see his 60-inch OLED screen over the round dome of his pannus, not quite contained by the too small T-shirt stained orange from his favorite flavor of nachos in the bowl on the end table next to him, on which also sits a half-squeezed tube of triple-antibiotic ointment that he intermittently applies to the chronic ulcer in the fragrantly-moist, smegma-coated skin-fold beneath his belly.

Your reality, good or bad, is a product of the choices you make, good or bad.

If you make a good choice you either increase the probability (Copenhagen) of a good outcome; or, you branch off into a parallel universe (Many Worlds) much more likely to have a good outcome.

Clearly, this applies to poor choices as well.

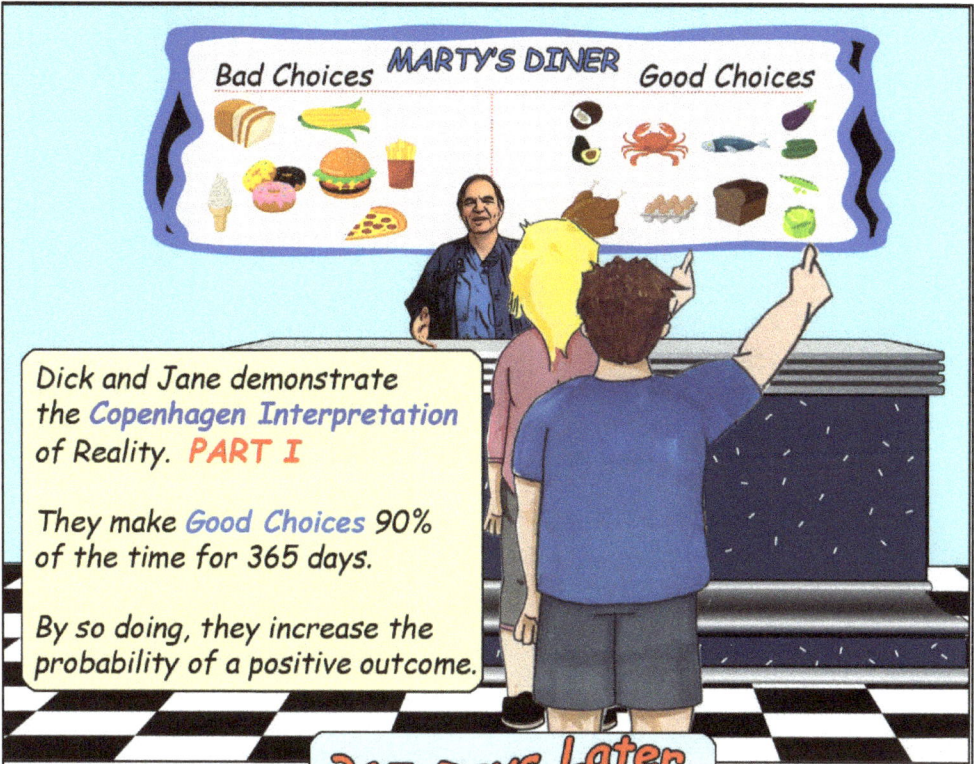

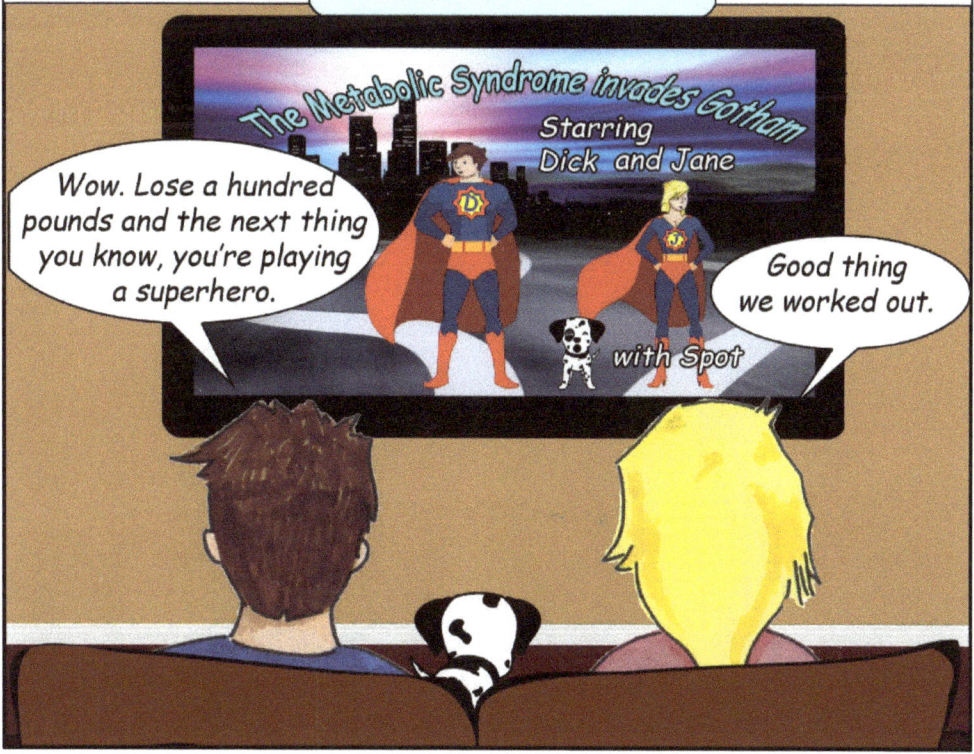

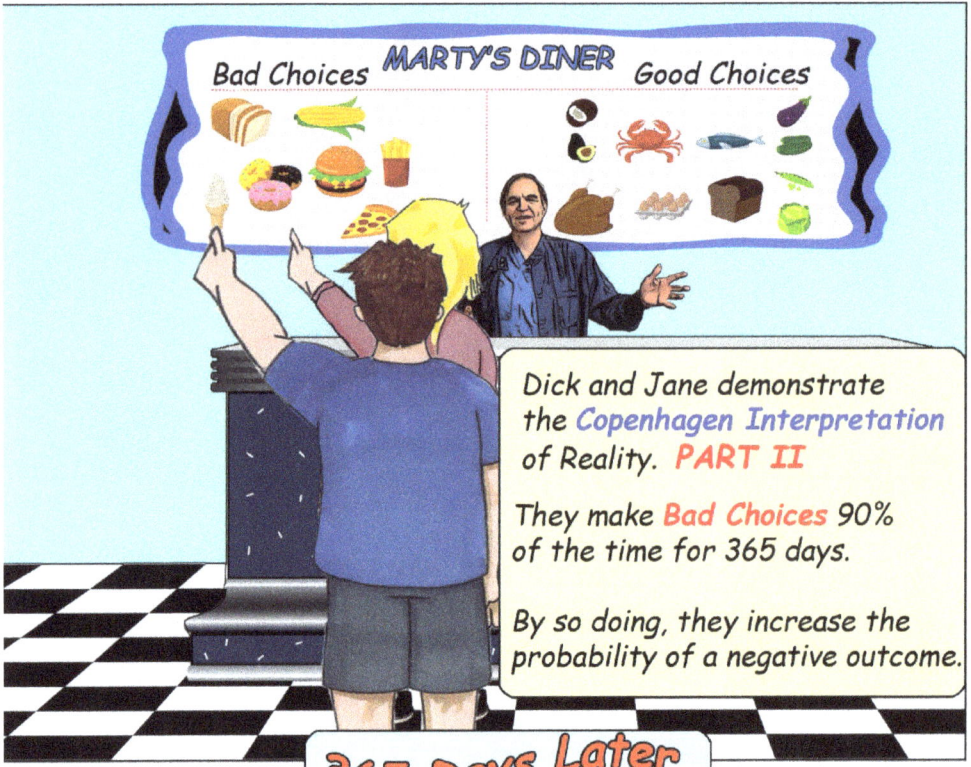

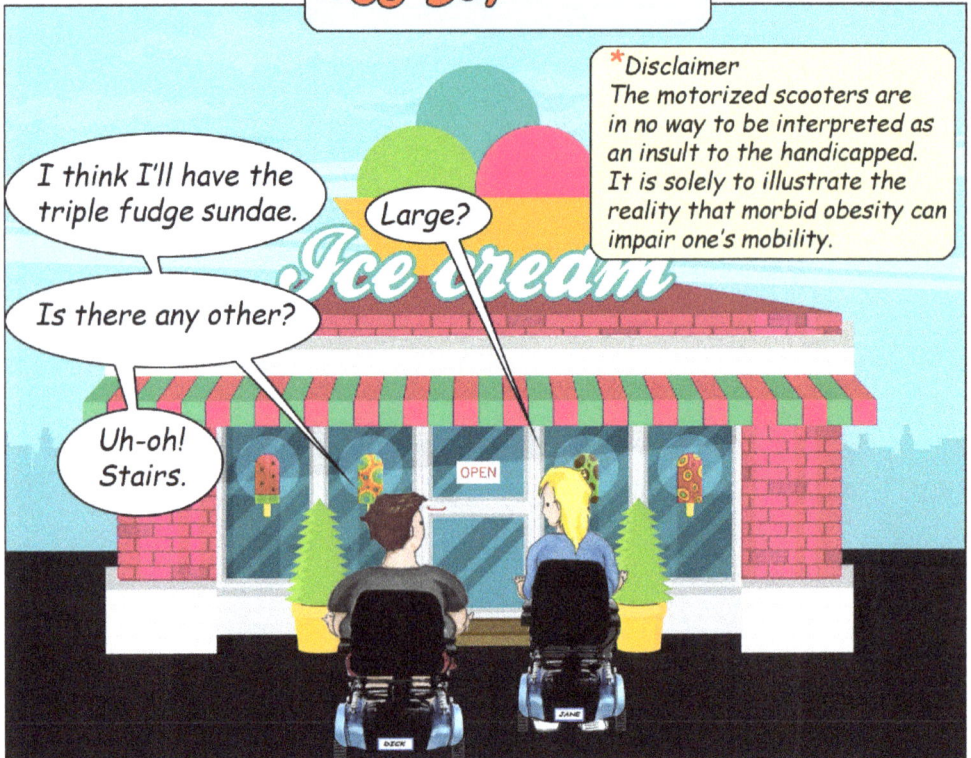

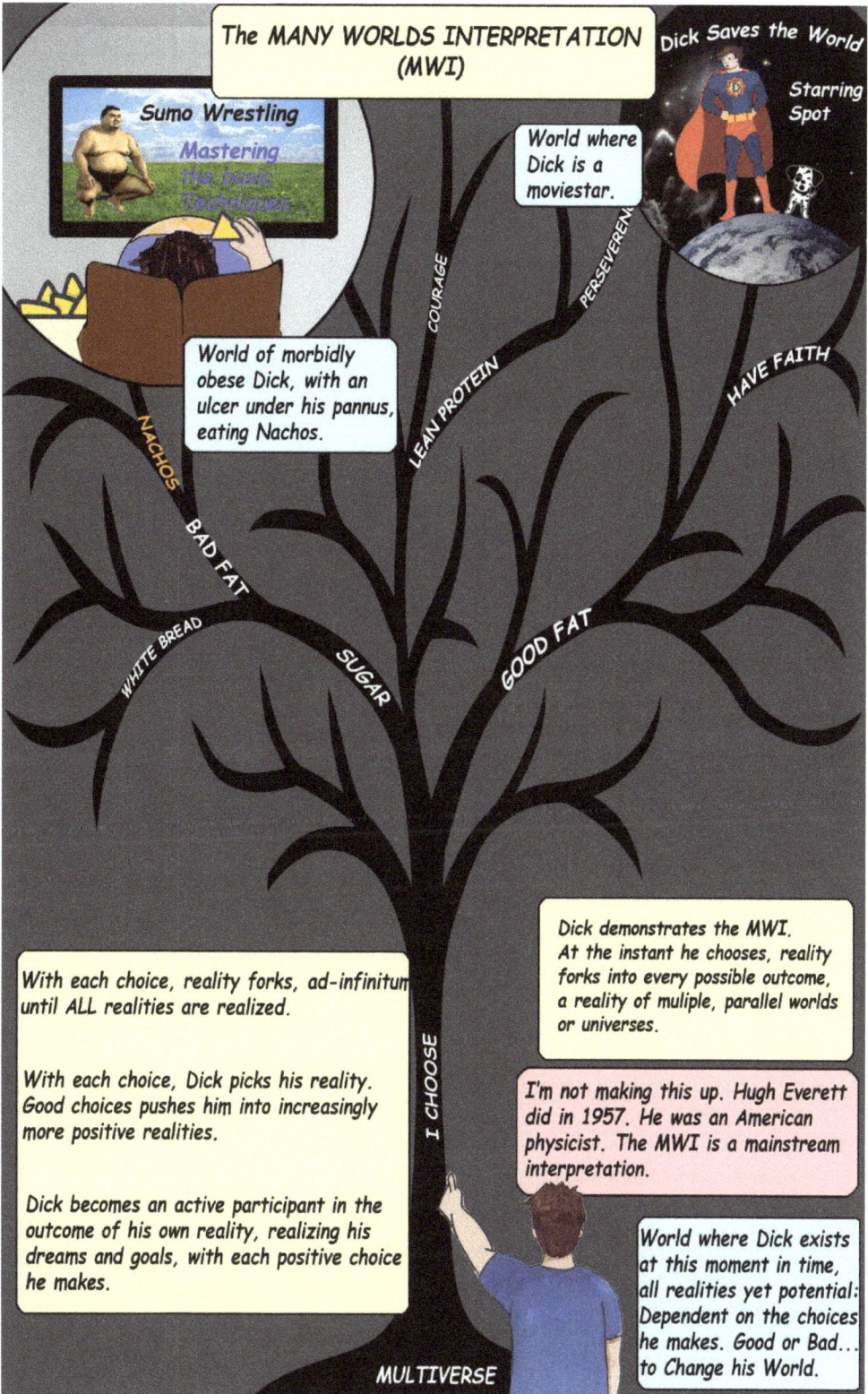

The MANY WORLDS INTERPRETATION (MWI)

Sumo Wrestling
Mastering the Basic Techniques...

Dick Saves the World
Starring Spot

World where Dick is a moviestar.

World of morbidly obese Dick, with an ulcer under his pannus, eating Nachos.

COURAGE

PERSEVEREN

LEAN PROTEIN

HAVE FAITH

NACHOS

BAD FAT

WHITE BREAD

SUGAR

GOOD FAT

Dick demonstrates the MWI. At the instant he chooses, reality forks into every possible outcome, a reality of muliple, parallel worlds or universes.

With each choice, reality forks, ad-infinitum until ALL realities are realized.

With each choice, Dick picks his reality. Good choices pushes him into increasingly more positive realities.

Dick becomes an active participant in the outcome of his own reality, realizing his dreams and goals, with each positive choice he makes.

I CHOOSE

I'm not making this up. Hugh Everett did in 1957. He was an American physicist. The MWI is a mainstream interpretation.

World where Dick exists at this moment in time, all realities yet potential: Dependent on the choices he makes. Good or Bad... to Change his World.

MULTIVERSE

Recognizing the universal truth of free will and the control you can exercise in the very selection of your own reality is one thing, making the proper choices is another, which leads to a final brief discussion of Sigmund Freud's psychoanalytical theory of personality, for therein lies potential tools and strategies to affect that very important process of changing your world by changing your thoughts, which we know are the root cause of the underlying pathology. Everyone has heard of the id, ego and superego, but most likely, the three are kind of mixed up as to the specific meaning, much less any practical application of the theory itself.

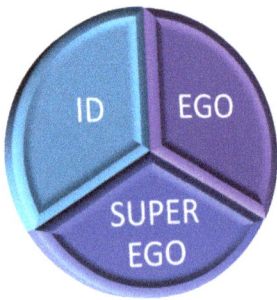

The three elements of Freudian personality form a trinity, almost like the Holy Trinity of the Father, the Son, and the Holy Spirit, representing three persons in one, except that I'm sure Sigmund did not feel similarly as he was a committed atheist to the suicidal end of his life. Nonetheless, like the Holy Trinity, the id, ego and superego represent three persons in one; the id is the only one present at birth, the ego comes online sometime after, and the superego by about the fifth year (17).

The id is primary. It is driven by the pleasure principle of immediate gratification for all wants and desires, without which a state of anxiety or tension builds within. The translation of id from Latin to English yields "it", and it wants. It wants warmth, food, drink, sex, soft things, shiny things. It is your inner animal, an animal without a conscience. In the spirit of making it sound less scary, **you might think of the id as your inner baby** that never grows up.

Unfortunately, our inner baby might metamorphose into an animal, like Dr. Jekyll into Mr. Hyde, a ravenous lustful selfish beast that must be tamed, which is where the ego and superego apply, the other two of the three persons of your trinity.

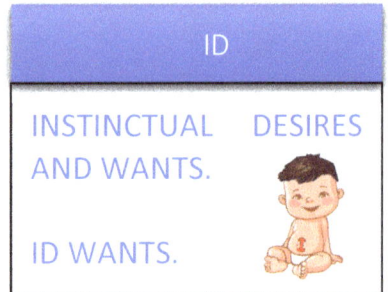

EGO
RESPONSIBLE; DEALS WITH REALITY. CONTROLS IMPULSES OF ID.

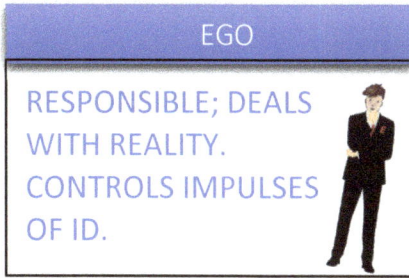

The ego is like your brake in the car on the road of reality. It is supposed to allow you to function in an acceptable fashion in the real world. It helps you delay your gratification or channel your behavior in a more appropriate fashion.

The third and final component of your trinity to develop is the superego. The superego represents your internalized moral standards that are acquired from your parents and society at large. It is your conscience, the voice over your shoulder whispering softly in your ear that only you can hear.

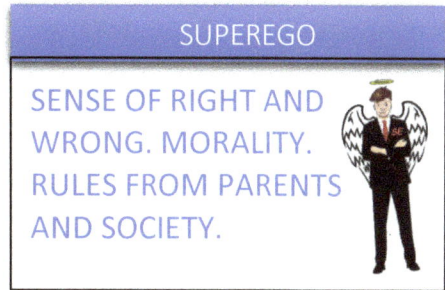

SUPEREGO
SENSE OF RIGHT AND WRONG. MORALITY. RULES FROM PARENTS AND SOCIETY.

I could pick anything. Believe me. In fact, it'd be more fun to pick something more risqué, but let's just play it safe and say we have a rum cake sitting on the counter. Your id loosens an instinctive primal urge in your mind so powerful it's as though it were a bevy of Odysseus's naked Sirens sitting on rocks outside the kitchen window, singing in shrill voices, "EAT IT! EAT IT NOW! EAT THE WHOLE #@$% THING! EAT IT. NOW!"

You find yourself in an internal three-way conversation, or you could say *battle*, between the id/ego/superego.

The Siren's screaming, "EAT IT. EAT IT. EAT IT. You know you want it. EAT! IT!"

Your ego squeaks, "Perhaps you should just have a piece, or else you'll be sick."

"Don't be stupid. It's pure poison," says your super ego with a frown (if it could frown). "God doesn't want you to eat any of it. It's wrong."

So, who's going to win that contest?

You.

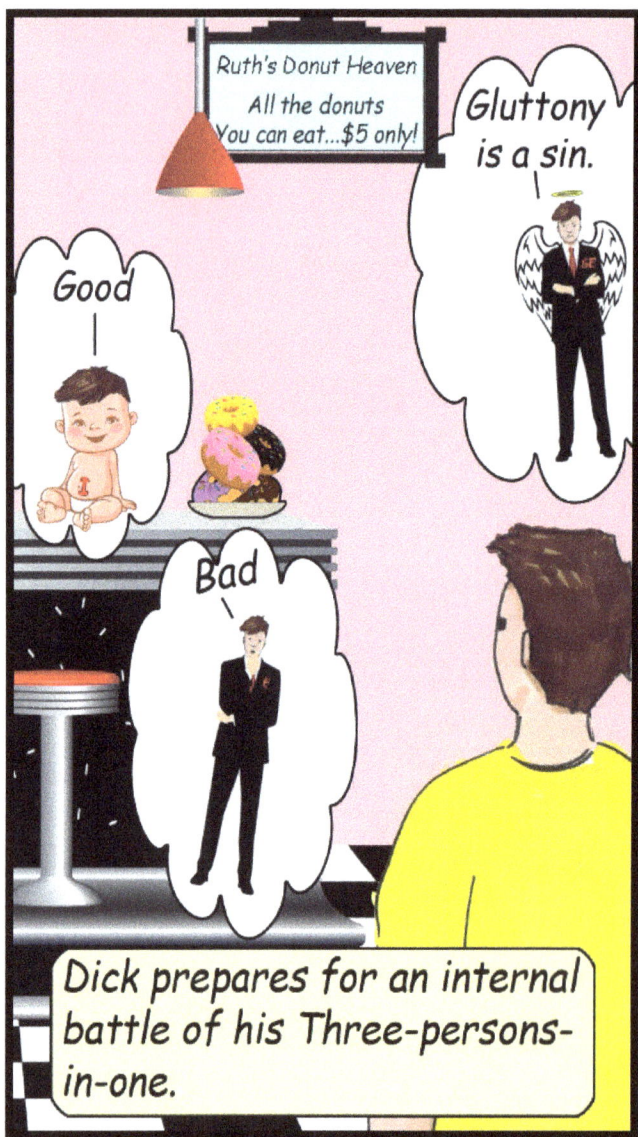

Good

Bad

Gluttony is a sin.

Ruth's Donut Heaven
All the donuts
You can eat...$5 only!

Dick prepares for an internal battle of his Three-persons-in-one.

You can win that contest by having an appreciation for the trinity that is you. You can separate the id from the ego, which is within the realm of truth and reality; and you can separate the id from the superego, which represents your conscience and sense of what is right and what is wrong, what is good and what is bad.

We can all recognize our inner baby. It wants…So, we acknowledge that desire for what it is. Now, it might be so bad that our ego stops it because the consequence of gratification might be a severe penalty, like not killing someone or else you'll go to prison for life or sit in the electric chair. In my personal case of the second occurrence of the chronic inflammatory condition from which I thought I was dying, the consequence of the gratification of my poor diet was the reality of death. The truth alone, as I felt it to be, was enough for my ego to apply the brake, to change my thoughts.

It is my hope that you might experience a similar success in the application of your own ego, when presented with the arrow of Truth, and change the way you've thought of food your entire life. In truth, it is difficult to completely separate the three as there is a harmony in the balance amongst them, and moderation of the id's desires is achieved by the application of reason and conscience by the ego and superego, respectively.

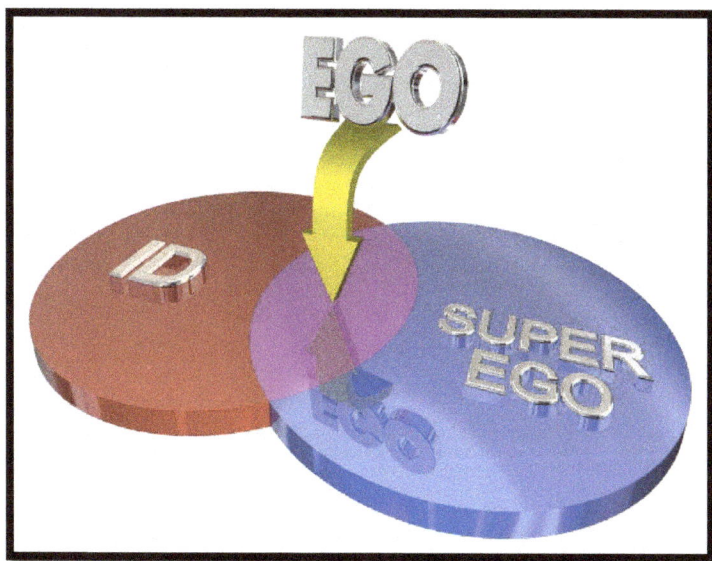

Will your ego and superego be able to control the desires of your inner animal, your inner baby? Well, that depends. It depends on which arrows you have in your quiver. Like I've said before, that's an easy one for me because I have the biggest, sharpest arrow of all. I have death, or at least the fear thereof, because, *right or wrong*, I've equated my chronic inflammatory pulmonary condition, and my ability to breathe, with obesity and the pro-inflammatory state that obesity engenders; and, the only thing I can do about it, other than take anti-inflammatory agents, is to affect some measure of control with my diet.

But that's not going to work for everybody, so we need more arrows and the first arrow, or strategy, is simply the Truth. The Truth of the caloric cost of the food that makes it to the dark side of your incisors. Possibly, perhaps, the truth alone shall set you free.

If you read the label, count the calories, record your daily intake in a journal or on a phone app like *Calorie Counter, My Plate, Lose It, My Fitness Pal*, etc.; if you make the effort to do those things, two things happen:

First, it takes time. It's like a buffer that allows your ego, and hopefully your superego (two are stronger than one) to overpower the Siren-call of your id. Secondly, once you know how many grams of sugar, how many calories that the ambrosia before you holds relative to the volume it represents; once you know the truth of that which your id wants to put inside you, I think the great majority of the time your egos will win because you will make a rational and moral decision that it is not worth it. Of course, there will be a rare instance, as ephemeral as the glowing tip of a sparkler fading to black on the 4th of July, like a frosty bottle of lager held out to you as you cross the finish line of the *Door County Triathlon*. Yes, an instant like that, when your id gets the last word *Oh, JUST DO IT!* and you do the math, and it's worth it.

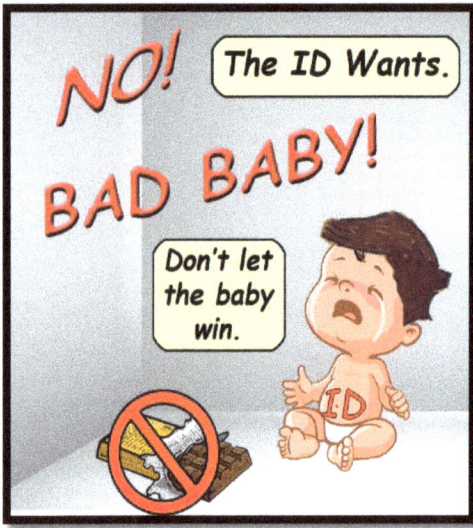

There you have it. The second arrow. *Reality.*

The *Copenhagen Interpretation* and *Many Worlds Interpretation* are both valid, current, scientific theories of reality, sharing the common theme of free will, and the power you hold within to control the outcome by making those choices that will manifest the reality you most desire. You can win the battle against your id by exercising your newly strengthened and reinforced ego and super ego. **Don't let the baby win.**

You literally have the power to build your own reality by making the choices that will either increase the probability of the reality you most desire occurring; or, by making the choices by which you will take successive forks down an infinitely branching reality of parallel universes until you end up on some yacht in the Mediterranean with a body-fat of less than 15% and either the Swedish Bikini team, or the male cast of *300*, parachuting in while you push away from your computer desk in the master cabin at the bow of the upper deck after selling the third batch of your bitcoin for a 2000% gain of some millions of dollars.

You now have two arrows; the arrow of Truth/Death, and the arrow of Reality/Free Will. In the next section, I will deliver the third and final arrow with which to slay the dragon of obesity. You are definitely almost a black belt now. I am excited for you.

Although the insinuation is that I am giving you the arrows, the truth is that you already have them. They are there. You have had them always. You only have to pick them up. I have had them my entire life, but only recently have begun to yield them more purposefully.

Lastly, you might have noticed that I hold a fondness for overdone, possibly slightly-grotesque, gratuitous-even, imagery. I assure you; it is mostly not autobiographical. I am the way I am for emphasis; using a sledge rather than a ball-peen hammer because I don't want to go, "chink, chink." I want to go **BAM, BAM.**"

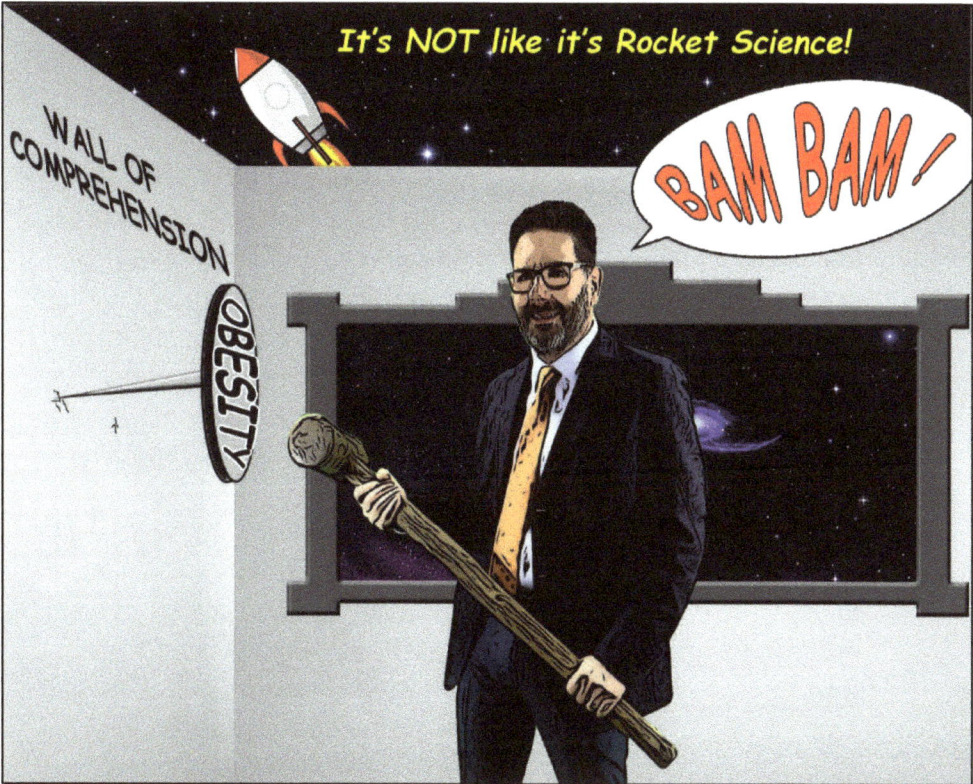

IT'S HAMMER-TIME!

It's like I'm a hammer and you're the nail. The wall of comprehension is thin and with each blow of the mighty hammer I am driving the sharp point of your intellect further and further into the wall that represents the barrier keeping you from that place you want to be. Deeper, deeper you go, realization dawning, leaking in like light through a crack in the clouds, until that happy moment when the point breaks through, the wall collapses, and you achieve weight loss enlightenment.

STRATEGIES FOR APPLYING FREUD'S TRINITY OF YOU.

1. **Acknowledge** your Id. Recognize it for what it is and what it wants, relative to your problem, in this case, obesity.
2. **Make a list of what id wants** that runs counter to your objective that you have in your home. The list should include all the foods that contain refined-sugar and complex carbohydrates like corn, rice, bread and pasta. It should also include unhealthy fats like commercial-grade (as opposed to grass-fed) red meat, processed meats like bacon and the trans-fats, as found in frozen pizza, doughnuts, fried fast foods, non-dairy coffee creamers, cakes, pies, cookies, frosting. The sources of trans-fats are generally so bad for you anyway that it is rather obvious.
3. **Remove** all the things on your list from your home. It is easier for your ego to say no to your id if they are not there.
4. **Make a list of the good foods** that your ego and superego want you to have to meet your objective. The list should include healthy sources of protein, like grass-fed beef, fish, free-range chicken and eggs; all vegetables that you like and would eat; good fats, like avocados, almonds, fish, coconut oil for cooking or a coconut powder coffee-creamer. Other better foods would be whole grains, squash and sweet potatoes (not with every meal). Dairy, like hard cheeses, Greek yogurt (no added sugar) and cottage cheese are safe foods.
5. **Replace** the things on the list in #2 with the things on the list in #4.

The above is redundant. You should already have done this in Phase I. It is the 2nd commandment; however, it is crucial and therefore warrants repetition. Perhaps rephrasing it in the recently cast light of Freud's psychoanalytical theory of the *ID/EGO/SUPEREGO* might cause you to think about it a little differently. This is purposeful on my part, *causing you to think about how you think.*

I want you to think about the appropriateness of your choices and to exercise *the power you hold* to exert some self-regulation and self-control. In the field of Cognitive Behavioral Therapy, this is a type of metacognition, which is a well-established therapeutic technique. "Meta" means *above or beyond*; and "cognition" means *thinking*. Cool. You've been metacognitized. Surprise.

Metacognition means *thinking how you think.*

When you see something you want, a cookie; that's your id.

When the voice says not to do it; that's your ego.

Free Will means you have the power to say no to yourself when you know something is wrong or bad for you.

This would be the appropriate time to introduce some ideas for stimulus control, utilizing the metacognitive aspects of your three-person-in-one. You need techniques/thoughts/ideas to control your inner baby. One list won't work for everybody because the most powerful techniques/thoughts/ideas are likely specific to each individual inner baby. This list is only limited by your imagination. It is important that you identify those specific to you and then to add to the list techniques/thoughts/ideas specific to you.

On the next page, I'll present an easy situation. There are much harder ones, ones that have nothing to do with dieting at all, but, with an awareness of your *inner-selves* should we say, you can hopefully *metacognate* (not a real word, but it fits) your way out of doing something utterly and completely stupid. All you have to do is *think about it*. You have to think about your motivators, your triggers, the bad things that can happen, and the good things if you do make the better choice to guide you into the reality you desire; then you need to establish actions, habits, techniques, thoughts with which you might counter such harmful tendencies.

Let me get you started…

Situation: You want to eat a rum cake, the whole damn thing, or at least until you get sick to your stomach. *What do you do?*

1. Stop. Think. How many calories is one serving? How big is one serving? Am I hungry? Am I angry, sad, bored? Why am I angry/sad/bored? *Is it worth it?*

2. Have a realistic or idealistic image of yourself as you would wish to be. This could be a picture from a time before you were overweight or obese if that ever was the case, or an image of another with the body habitus you'd like to achieve. Have it in your mind. You might have it in an inside cupboard at home, or in your wallet or purse or on your phone, but at least have it in your mind. Imagine it. *Is it still worth it?*

3. *Say a short prayer, like the Hail Mary, or a motivational verse or quote.*

4. Think of the ingredients as poison, the combination of bad fats and sugar; the accompanying surge of insulin; the storage of fat; fat like the glistening translucent whorls cut from a fatty steak being stored in your body.

5. Pinch your sub-cutaneous tissue to either side of your belly button. How thick is it? *Is it still worth it?*

6. Close your eyes, blink, turn away, give yourself some positive affirmation. I am loved. I am a good person. I can do this for myself. I choose a different reality. I choose a different universe. *Is it still worth it?*

7. Leave. If you're in the breakroom, take the time to do any of the above or equivalent while you're leaving.

8. If you succumb, all is not lost. Yet. With that first bite of whatever it is, does it taste as good as you imagined it would, or is it stale, rather tasteless? How good is it, really? *Is it still worth it?*

9. *...you are only limited by your imagination.*

The above are all rather simple techniques for when you are exposed to the bait of the dragon inadvertently. Remember, this shouldn't happen inside your castle, outside of the holidays with visiting family and friends, when there tends to be bait all over the place, in which case you'll find yourself saying a lot of prayers, pinching yourself, blinking, and possibly inducing mild nausea from gross mental imagery having to do with fat and your **WAT** gland.

There is much more that you can do, much more that you should do, more mindful things; however, I will be addressing those in the next section, the Arrow of Belief.

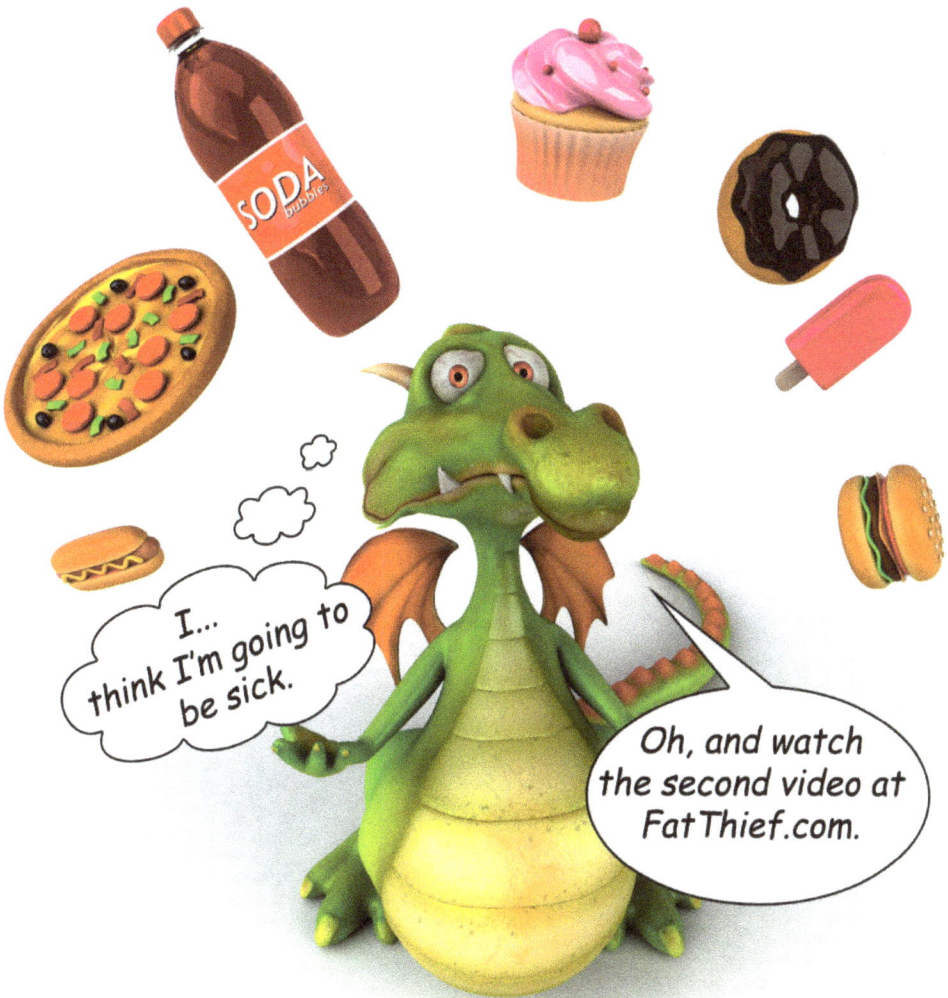

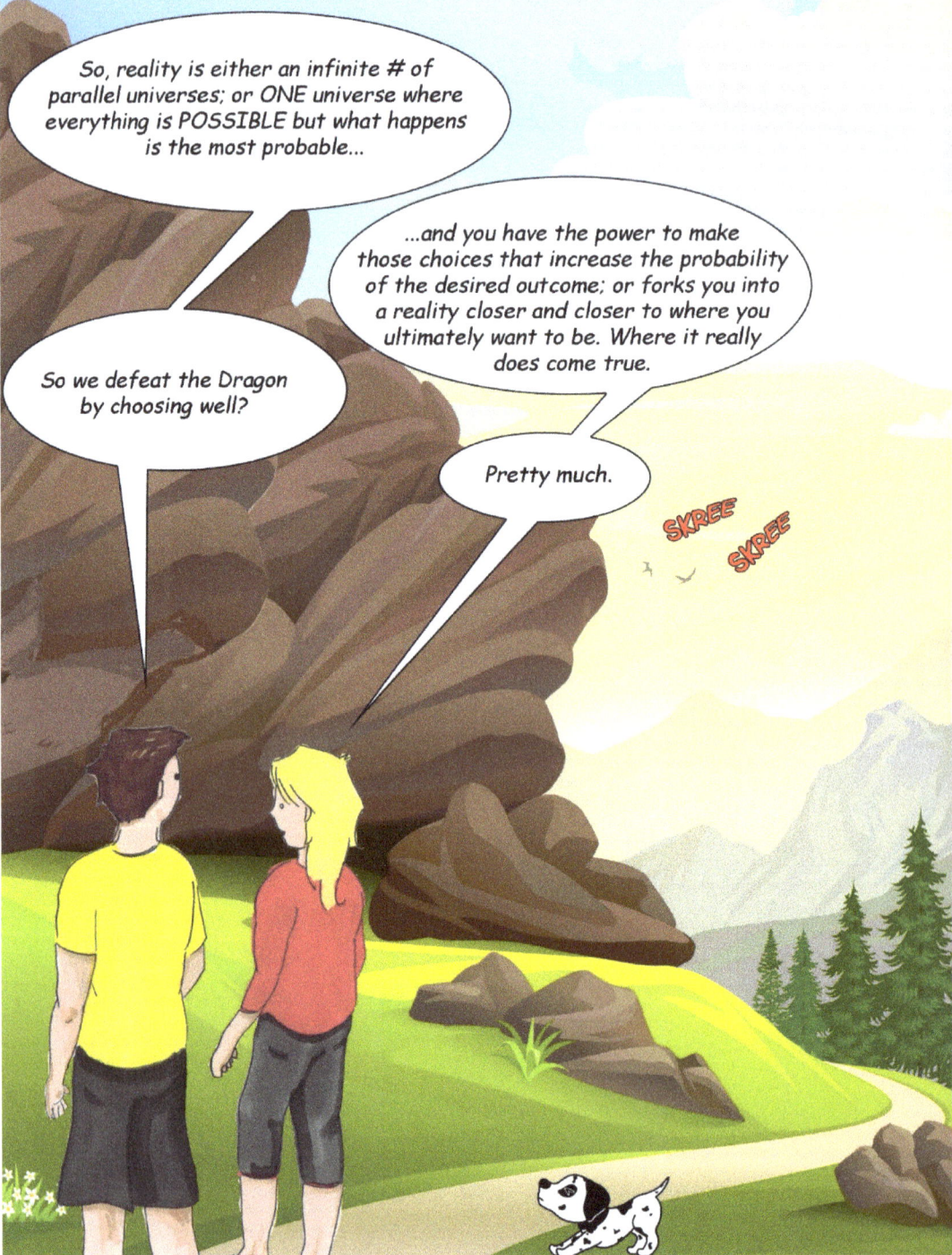

Dick and Jane have covered much ground on their Allegorical quest. Yet, there is more they must do. Although the end approaches, it is more the end of the beginning.

So, reality is either an infinite # of parallel universes; or ONE universe where everything is POSSIBLE but what happens is the most probable...

...and you have the power to make those choices that increase the probability of the desired outcome; or forks you into a reality closer and closer to where you ultimately want to be. Where it really does come true.

So we defeat the Dragon by choosing well?

Pretty much.

SKREE

SKREE

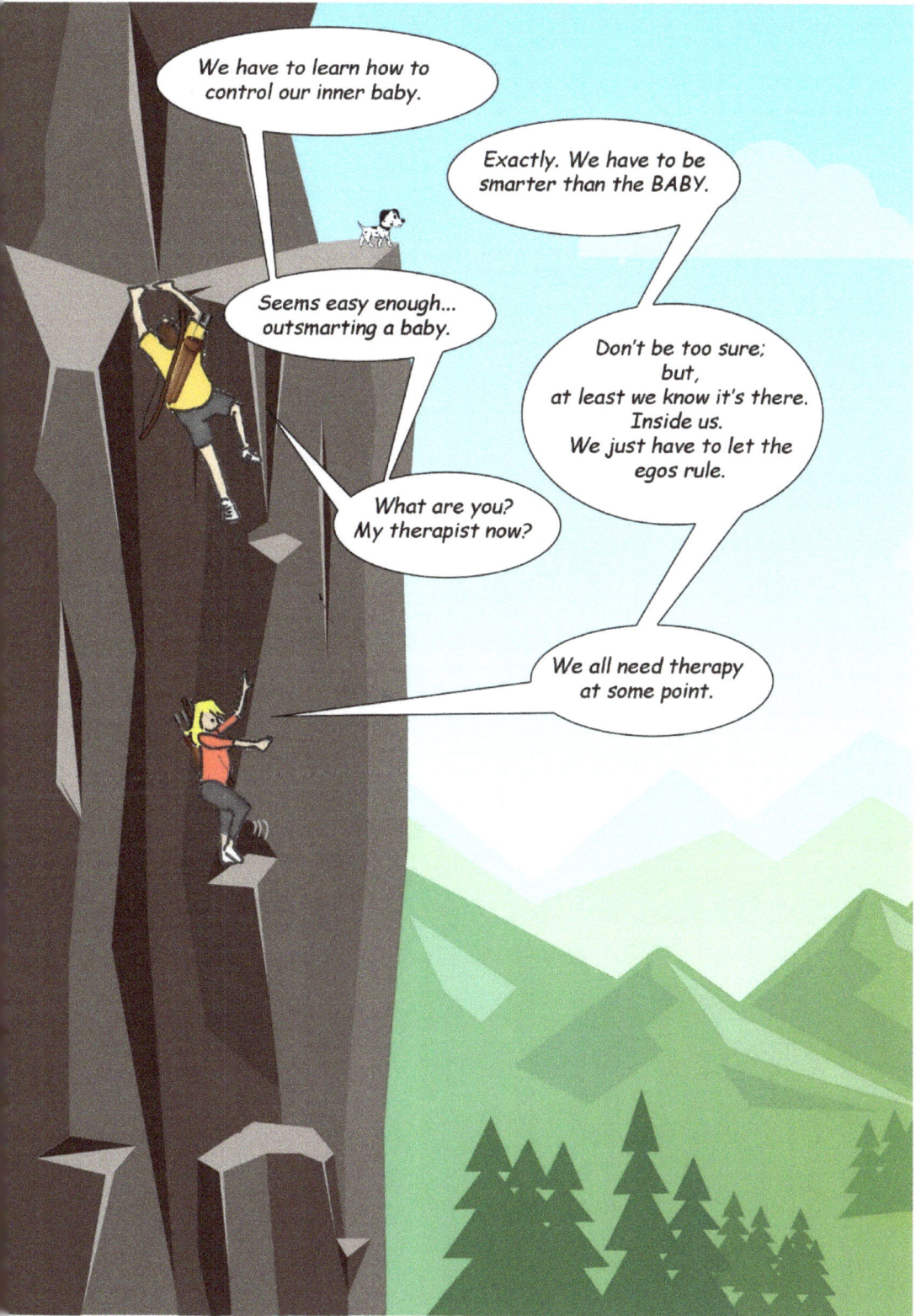

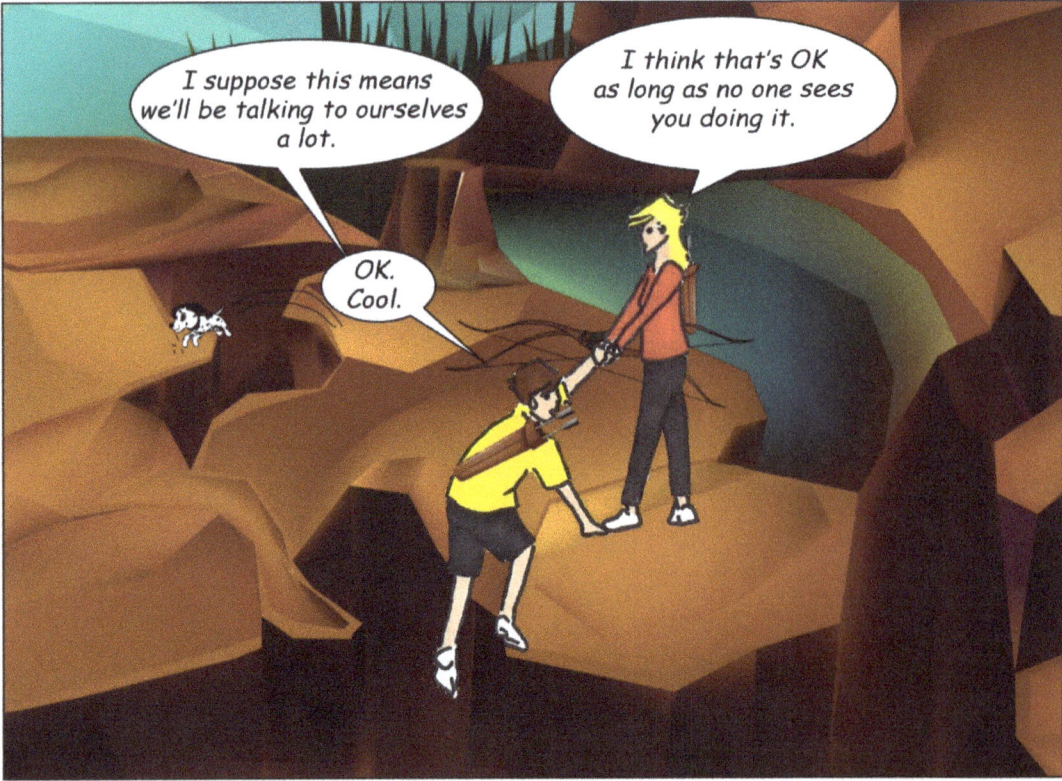

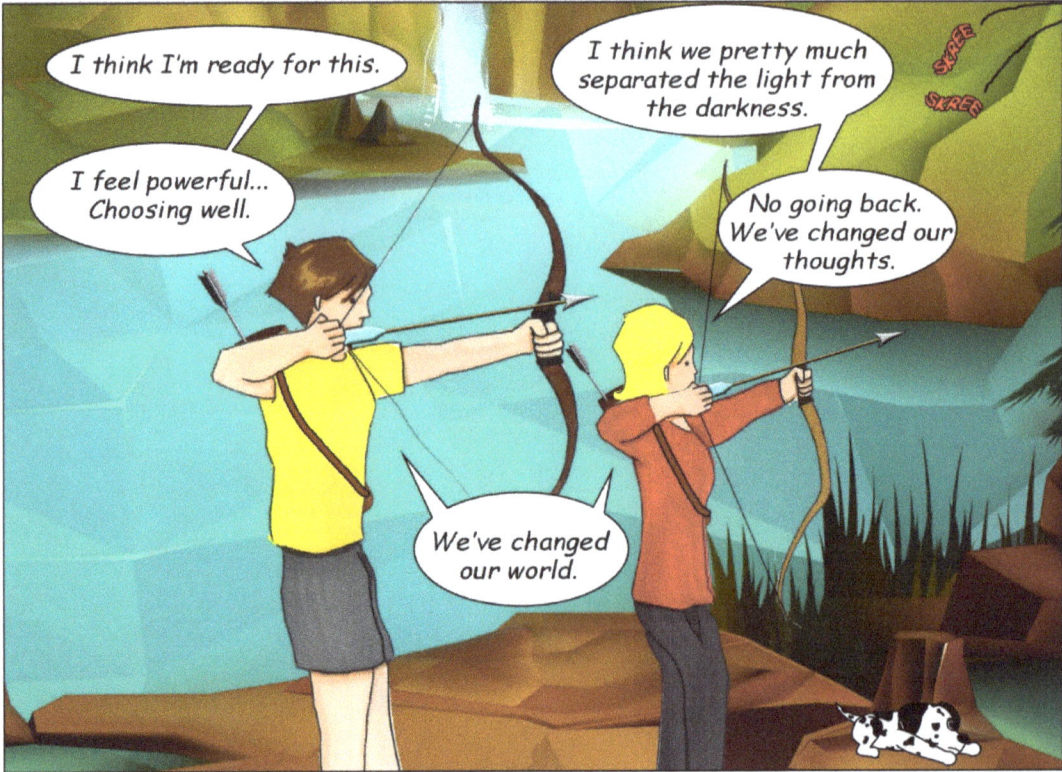

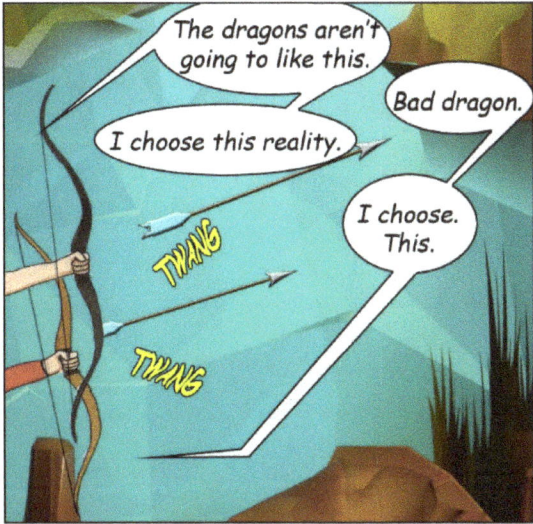

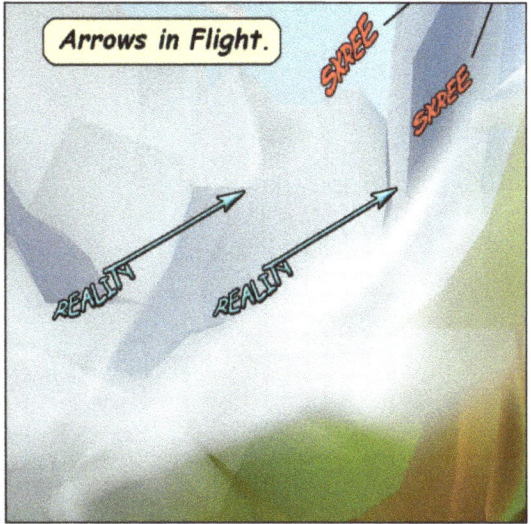

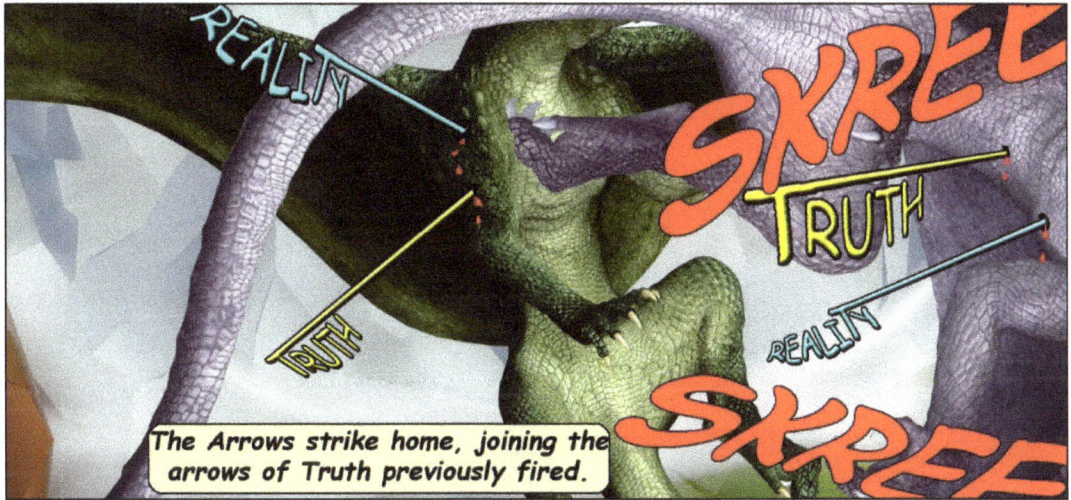

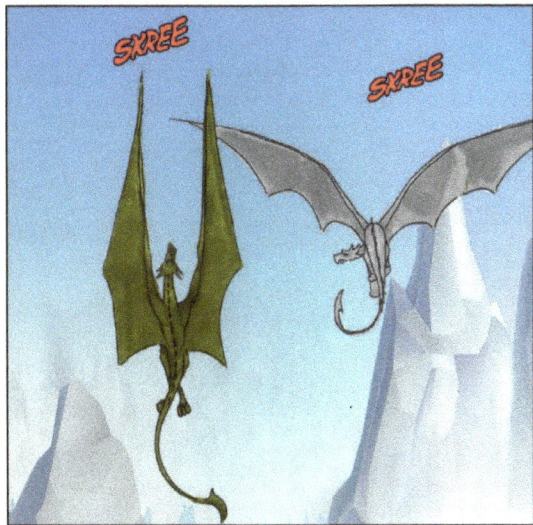

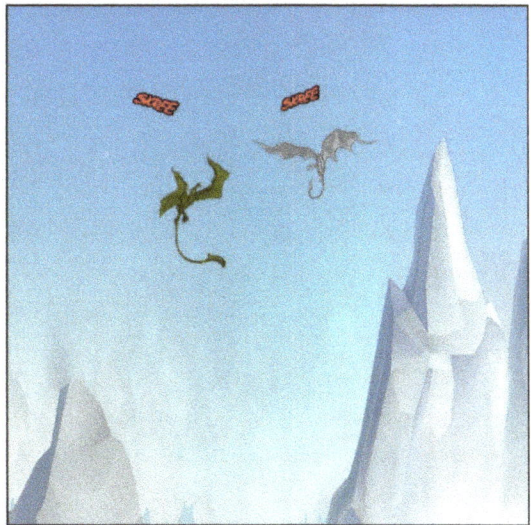

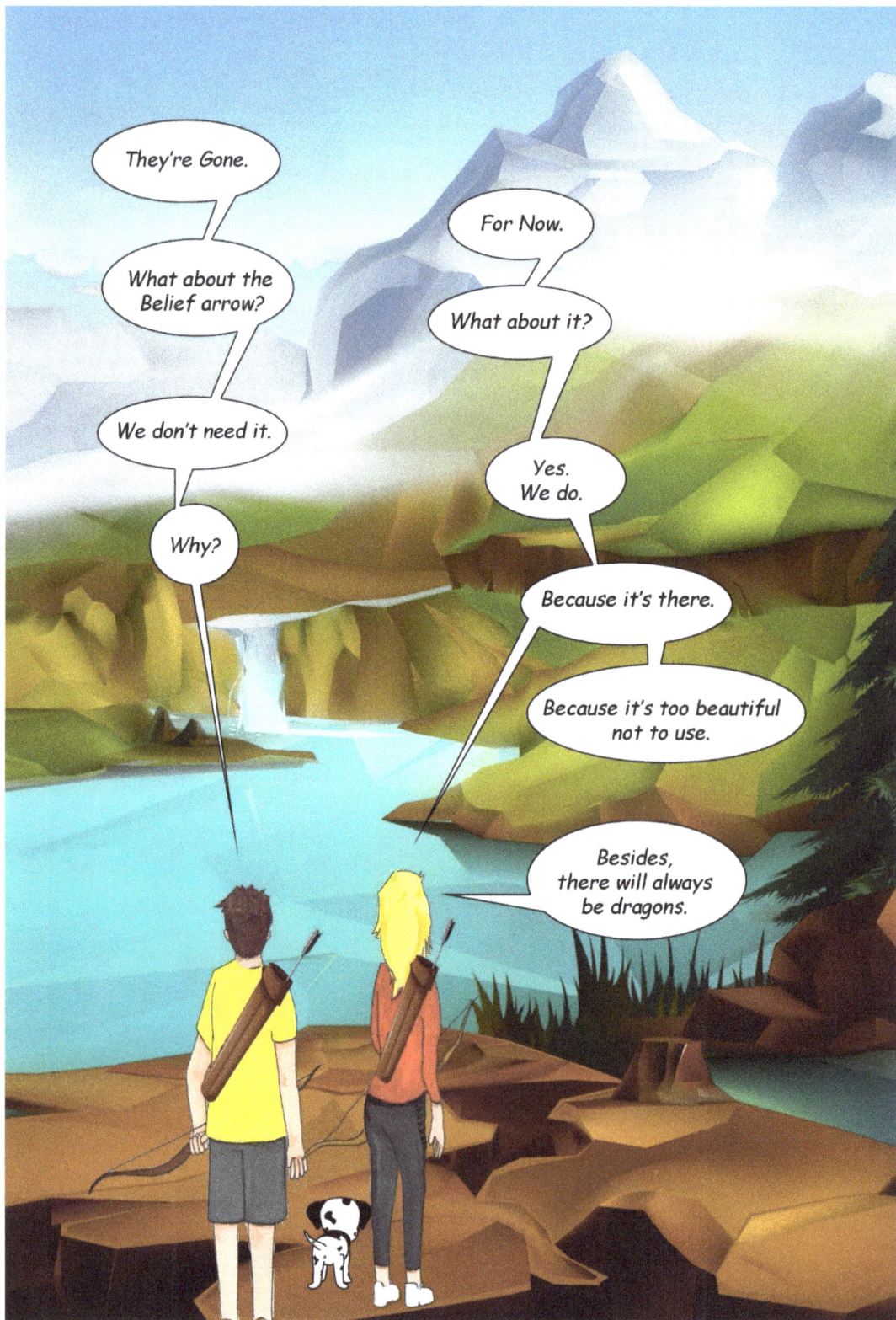

BELIEF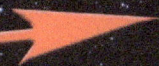

BEHOLD.

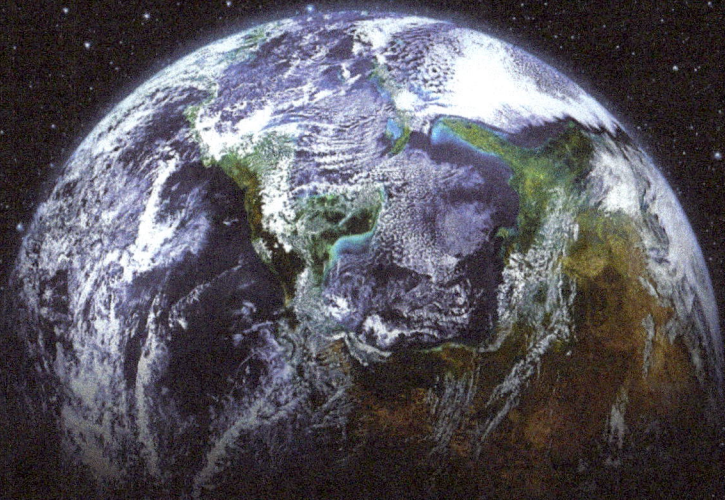

CHAPTER EIGHT: Belief: First Component

In my attempts to impart strategies and tools by which you might positively affect your own behavior I have chosen this motif of "arrows." Arrows that you might pull from an imaginary quiver on your back, like Katniss Everdeen in the Hunger Games, or a Mongol racing on horseback across the steppes of central Asia during the Tang Dynasty.

The *first arrow* was that of *Truth*: the truth about the three primary macronutrients (fats, carbs, protein) and how the indiscriminate use thereof might result in illness and death. The *second arrow* was that of *Reality*: how the reality you are living is the direct result of the choices you make, and the relative power you have to select the reality you wish to inhabit.

Now, I wish to impart to you a *third arrow*, the arrow of *Belief*. I should again clarify that I am not giving you these arrows. You already have them in your quiver. You've had them your entire life. These words are only my attempt to illustrate that which already exists.

There are two components to the Belief arrow as I see it. The thing is, I've spent over a hundred and twenty pages, telling you that you have the power to literally change your world by choosing well, and that by doing so you will select your own reality. You will create, with your choices, the universe you want to live in.

Well. Life is still hard. It's not going to be easy all the time. There will be times when you make the right choices and bad things still happen, those times when things don't seem fair; but, the sheer weight of continued positive actions, positive thoughts, positive choices will overcome all. I believe that to be inevitable. But; to do this, to do all these things, being an active participant in this world in which you find yourself, requires much. It requires courage, conviction, confidence; it requires dedication, perseverance, resilience; and for all that to happen, you must believe in yourself. You must believe that you can do this, and that is the first component of the Belief arrow, a belief in yourself.

The second component is of a spiritual nature that some may not be interested in pursuing, and that is fine. My purpose is to help all those who need help, regardless of belief systems; however, if you are a spiritual person, I believe that your faith in a power higher than yourself should be an integral part in the self-selection of your reality.

The 12-Step Program of Alcoholics Anonymous was established in 1939 and became an accepted and well-known strategy that is broadly used in the treatment of many addictions.

The First Three Steps of Alcoholics Anonymous

1. We admitted we were powerless over alcohol—that our lives had become unmanageable.
2. Came to believe that a Power greater than ourselves could restore us to sanity.
3. Made a decision to turn our will and our lives over to the care of God as we understood Him.

If you believe in God, He should be a significant part of your world, and your recovery from obesity.

In truth, greater than 90% of the behavioral strategies and techniques I'll be discussing are not faith-based, but that does not mean that the spiritual component of the Belief Arrow is not important. Quite the contrary, and I save this for the very end, for those who would like to travel that road. To those so inclined to read all the way to the end, you might say, *I saved the best for last.*

> Fast digesting carbohydrates, like those in sweets and soda, stimulate the same areas of brain involved in addictive behavior.

Like alcohol and drugs, food *can* be like an addiction too. In fact, fast-digesting carbohydrates (refined sugar) have been shown to stimulate the same areas of the brain involved in addictive behavior (18). Like alcohol and drugs and other things, over-eating becomes a pattern of behavior, if not an addiction. The frustrating truth is that most everyone, at the very basic level, knows what to do. They know what they should eat. They know they should eat less and exercise more and so on; but most everyone still doesn't do it for whichever reason.

To break a pattern of behavior requires a modification of that behavior or those behaviors. The patterns of behavior are established by what feels good, what tastes good, basically, whatever satisfies the *pleasure principle* which drives the id, your inner baby. You like it, *id* wants, and so you do it; therefore, to not do it requires a self-denial of sorts. It requires daily sacrifice, even if on a small scale.

Sacrifice. Saying no to the id, your inner baby. Denial. delayed gratification, patience, behavioral modification strategies you employ are some of the forms your sacrifice might take.

> The daily sacrifices that you make for your better good becomes the primary way for you to lose weight, or pretty much accomplish anything else you wish to do in this world.

I want you to think of how others have sacrificed. Young men and women in our military forces who gave of themselves so that others may live; all the men and women in public service, firemen, policemen; good Samaritans stepping into harm's way, like those young men on the train in Paris who disarmed a terrorist, running towards the AR-15 that misfired.

These examples represent the supreme sacrifice of self, or the potential sacrifice of self; however, there are many other examples of those who give of themselves in other ways; a parent working two jobs or late into the nights so that you might have a bike to ride or new clothes for school; a close friend who gave something up for you, covered a shift, took on an extra burden for your sake; an unknown person who bought you a meal as a surprise or the stranger ahead of you in the drive-thru at Starbucks who paid for your coffee. It is in our nature to sacrifice, to offer ourselves for the greater good, for your fellow man, for God, for Country. It's about time that you sacrifice for yourself.

I believe the first step towards breaking a harmful pattern of behavior would be at the beginning, or at any point along the way, to retreat to a quiet place for a quiet period of contemplation or meditation where you reflect on where you are relative to where you want to be.

Recognize that you have been powerless or unable to make the necessary choices and that you need help. Your first source of help is of course yourself. You are reading this manual. You are learning. This might be enough; however, you may need more. This requires some quiet time and deep thought.

You must break your patterns of behavior that are harmful towards your goal of losing weight. How do you do that? How do you affect a modification in those behaviors? *First, you must establish a beginning.*

> It is important to SET A START POINT. A time in your life that you can look back on, a point in time that separates what was before from what came after.

This first step could happen anywhere; a quiet place on a quiet day in your backyard, at your church, on a partly sunny spring day on the edge of a bluff, sitting in the lotus position as you overlook the blue expanse of Lake Michigan. You need think about where you are and where you want to be. You need to find your resolve, to say to yourself *I can do this. I am ready for this.*

Maybe you've already done this, or some version thereof. If not, it's never too late. It's important to mark a start point, a memory of that point in time that you decided to change your world, a day and a place you long remember. That is just the beginning. You, I, we, as creatures of habits, need more, because simply thinking it won't make it come true. We need action. We need to participate emotionally, physically, wholeheartedly, enthusiastically.

We need daily reminders and new habits, new patterns of behavior to combat the old for we are only human, all too human. No saints are we. We are weak and overly prone to succumbing to our inner baby, the id. So, what are some additional strategies or coping mechanisms we might apply?

Remember, there is the arrow of Truth and the arrow of Reality/Free-Will; however, we are considering some additional strategies to modify our behaviors relative to the Belief arrow; strategies that are more mindful, strategies that are a degree of magnitude of greater significance than the more utilitarian techniques/thoughts/ideas previously discussed.

Presented on the following page is a list of strategies that is not inclusive. There is nothing magical about it. These are things that have been helpful for me and to many others. The important thing is to start with something, even if only one thing, or two. You should be able to make your own additions to the list that are specific to you, that will help you make those choices that you know are right, but struggle with all the same.

A Suggested List of Strategies

---

1.   Identify those core beliefs and assumptions that are faulty or distorted.

Core beliefs are foundational beliefs that form the essence of you as you know yourself. They are formed early in childhood. A false core belief would be something like *nobody loves me. I am worthless. I am meaningless. I do not matter.*

This is primary. You *need to be healthy inside*, and by that, I mean to say that you need to have a positive self-image. If you can look at yourself in the mirror and honestly say and feel, *I love, I am loved, I am a good person*, then you should be fine; however, if there is any doubt, you must do more that is beyond the scope of this manual. I would suggest asking your primary care provider for a referral to Behavioral Therapy for a well-defined professional approach. This is something that would be in conjunction with living a healthy lifestyle, including diet, as you are learning of in these pages before you.

If you would rather explore your core beliefs and assumptions on your own initially, further action could include the utilization of a specific workbook that uses the tool of thought records or thought journaling. One such book that has been around for many years and can help you with this is *Mind Over Mood* (19).

For you to wield your arrow of belief you must have healthy core beliefs. You must respect yourself. You must have love in your heart; this you need for that first component of belief, or belief in self. I do believe this is easier for a spiritual person for the simple reason that if you believe in God, and God is Love, well, then...

Again, if you think your core beliefs might be faulty, please seek additional help.

---

2. Start each day with a meditation or prayer.

Perhaps, first thing in the morning, when you awake, before opening your eyes: A prayer meaningful to you such as the Serenity prayer of AA; a goal for the day, a positive affirmation of yourself; appreciation for something.

I love my life. I am a good person. Life is beautiful. My life is precious. Thank you for my life.

---

3. Go to your church, or special place, regularly.

Use that time to reflect on the day/week past and the day/week to come relative to your goals and objectives; quiet your mind; be still. Try to be still for at least thirty minutes. No talking.

---

4. Acquire a talisman.

The definition of which is *an object held to act as a charm to avert evil and bring good fortune*. However, rather than a mere charm, assign it more significance. This could be of a religious significance (a blessed medal); or an item associated with the significance of a commitment made to yourself or another, or your Higher Power.

> An example of a talisman would be a special necklace, ring, bracelet, medal, or similar that you can wear, which serves as a physical reminder of your commitment to your purpose.

A talisman could be a relic of sorts, something passed down from your family, something important to you. If there is no such thing, find something, buy something, then *make it important to you*. This could be a bracelet, ring, necklace; something that you *wear at all times*.

You need to remember it and why you wear it. You can feel it, touch it, and remember why you wear it, and you might think to yourself *I can do this*.

A talisman is a useful coping mechanism. It can serve as a physical reminder of your purpose in this world, or a purpose. We already have these things that are precious to us: a small metal statue you were given as a child, an old photo of a loved one no longer with you, a ring or watch or necklace from a parent or grandparent or close friend, a music box with a spinning ballerina from your grandmother. Find something small and wearable, or something you might see every day. Most likely you already have such a thing.

Assign the value of your commitment to it in prayer or meditation; then, wear it, see it. Always. Feel it on your skin, against your chest or on a finger or wrist. It will become some source of comfort and resolve in some small measure as you negotiate your day. See it on the top shelf in your locker at work, on your dresser in the bedroom. Every day.

It might even acquire magical properties, like turning warm in warning in passing a display case of pastries; or, maybe you'll find that when you touch the cinnamon roll, it, like the Holy Water splashed on Linda Blair in *The Exorcist*, burns your skin.

It could happen. It probably does happen in some alternate reality, in some parallel universe somewhere. Put physical reminders on display in places of weakness (kitchen) and strength (bedroom, office, exercise room).

Hang a physical reminder from a small adhesive hook stuck to the front of the fridge that is impactful to you. If it's something strange, like a fat voodoo doll with a pin sticking out of the belly, I'd suggest taking it down before company comes over, especially if you're single and it's a date night.

A physical reminder could also be a favorite inspirational quote, a picture, a religious icon. An example of a quote would be like this one from the Dalai Lama:

"To conquer oneself is a greater victory than to conquer thousands in a battle."

You need to identify something that has value and is meaningful for you. In your places of strength, display motivational quotes or pictures that make you feel positive and good, physical reminders that you matter, are loved, and are worthy.

I've learned that people will forget what you said, people will forget what you did, but people will never forget how you made them feel.

–Maya Angelou

---

5. As you would have a physical talisman, you should have a mental talisman as well, what would be considered a mantra.

This could be a short, meaningful prayer or quote, or a traditional Eastern mantra. Some popular mantras that I like, especially the last one, are:

"Love is the only miracle there is." *Osho*
"Be the change you wish to see in the world." *Gandi*
"Every day in every way I am getting better and better." *Laura Silva*
"I change my thoughts, I change my world." *Norman Vincent Peale*

You use your mental talisman during times of stress, when your id is screaming in your ear. You breathe deep, and whisper or see the words in your mind. Anything works. You can find a biblical quote or passage or research a traditional Eastern mantra. It helps if it is short, less than ten syllables; and it helps if you can feel it when you say it, like drawn out vowel sounds (Aaaa, Eeee, Oooo, Eye) and consonants that you feel in your chest (mmmm,nnnn).

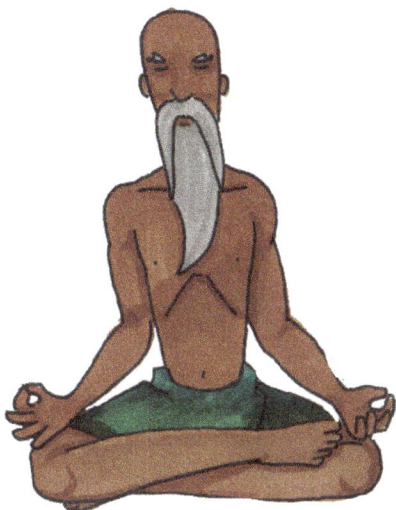

You don't have to be in the lotus position to use a mantra. You use it anywhere, anytime, in any position.

REFER TO APPENDIX K FOR FUTHER HELP WITH MANTRAS

6. Harness the power of social support.

The first four strategies are contemplative and solitary. For many people, if not most, a social support structure is very helpful. This is why weight-loss contests, usually after the holidays are so popular, and often effective.

Joining an online diet group through Facebook or other social networks is only one thing you could do. Enlisting the support of your healthcare network, your primary care provider, a Behavioral Management consult, if necessary, are things that may be covered by insurance. Embarking on your weight-loss journey lifestyle change might be done with a spouse, a friend or group of friends. The point is to not do it alone. Rather, you do it together. There are online communities and phone apps, such as Noom; however, many of these do have monthly costs.

There's over a 100 million people in our country who are struggling with their weight. You don't have to be alone. In fact, you shouldn't be alone. The consensus medical opinion is that a social support network plays a vital role in your weight-loss efforts and in the maintenance of weight loss.

You should first seek support close to home, a spouse and/or other family members or a group of like-minded friends. If you are following a specific diet strategy, such as a ketogenic or plant-based strategy, then search for online communities that follow those strategies. Facebook, Instagram, Twitter are the obvious. Form a Facebook or Outlook group or a Google circle of your own if you are so inclined.

> **PLEASE REFER TO THE APPENDIX I FOR A LIST OF ONLINE WEIGHT-LOSS COMMUNITIES.**

7. Start a Journal or a Blog

A powerful motivator as well as a tremendous support can be a record of your thoughts. A journal is traditional, old school. A blog is new school, easy and free. Just because it's in the cloud, available for anyone to see on the world wide web, does not mean that it will be seen. It is completely up to you. It can be a private record that only you can unlock, or you can share it with a select few, or the world.

The convenience of a blog is what makes it special. It is always there. You know where it is, as long as you remember the password. You can write in it at home, at work, on vacation, anywhere you have an internet connection and a phone, laptop or computer. This is what many people have done, not necessarily for weight loss, but for things that they care about and want to share. Sometimes a blog will strike a common chord in a community of like-minded souls and it will take off and grow beyond all expectations.

I did this for a few months when I was sick. It was anonymous, private and available for the world to see, but few did. I figured that when I died, it would go away, lapse, and I found comfort in the idea of it and the indulgent expression of my innermost thoughts.

It is so easy to start a blog that there is no reason not to do it. It is as important to have the support of others as it is to support others as it is to support yourself. Writing is only one way to accomplish that.

I will have an online presence for the purpose of offering additional support at *FatThief.com*. It is important that you remain engaged during this process of changing your world, and I can help you with that. In addition to the base materials at the site, I will be posting additional articles, links and videos that will be of interest and of help to you.

> **START A JOURNAL OR A BLOG.**
>
> **PLEASE REFER TO THE APPENDIX J FOR A LIST OF FREE BLOG SITES.**

This itemized list of seven is just the beginning, and it will be different for different people. I only stopped at seven because it's lucky.

You must find what works for you, what gives you strength, what gives you resolve and determination and perseverance. That is your task, to identify those things and then to utilize those things in your coping strategies.

In a parallel universe where the inhabitants speak only in Haiku verse with a sporadic iambic pentameter overlay.

.

*I have a confession to make, but it is not a sin. It is a good thing, but I can only tell you here at the end because only now will you appreciate the impact. As I said at the very beginning, the primary focus of this effort is to get you to change your thoughts so that you can change your world. Well, that requires some therapy. Up to the 1950's, Freud's psychoanalysis was prevalent; however, subsequent to that, Cognitive Behavioral Therapy (**CBT**) has been dominant although variants of both are practiced today (26)*

Cognitive Behavioral Therapy (CBT) is a type of psychotherapy treatment helpful for the treatment of many psychological illnesses. It consists of talk therapy, setting goals and problem-solving with the purpose of changing negative patterns of thought and/or behaviors that are the source of the patient's difficulties.

I didn't want to write a diet book or instructional manual with the primary focus of telling you what to do, and then hoping that you do it. I wanted more than that. I wanted to, in effect, operate on your brain, but not with a scalpel; rather, with the blades of logic, reason and belief. An operation to resect, modify or repair those dysfunctional thoughts and assumptions that are leading to dysfunctional behaviors, negatively impacting your diet and health. In this process, I have followed specific steps that have been well defined by CBT models.

THE STEPS OF CBT THAT YOU HAVE ALREADY DONE OR WILL DO

1. IDENTIFY THE PROBLEM

You identified the problem: *I am overweight or obese.* There is a reason for that. It may be secondary to dysfunctional beliefs about what you should eat or the amount, which may be as simple as a carelessness with the macronutrients you eat, or it may be more complex. It may be that you have destructive thoughts about your self-worth *how could anyone like me*; your body-image *I'm hopelessly fat*; your potential *I'm stuck and will never amount to anything*; or, it could be as serious as a false core belief.

Severe pathology in dysfunctional automatic thinking or core belief systems is beyond the scope of a book. Professional counseling, both individual and group would be of benefit, if not required. If you feel that to be even remotely a possibility in your case, please ask your primary care provider for a referral for professional guidance.

2. SET GOALS

You set goals: You identified an appropriate BMI for yourself. You selected a palatable dietary strategy to implement from the spectrum presented. *Phase I/commandments 1,3*

You recognize the importance of accountability, exercise and sleep and know that you must be responsible and take care of yourself.

3. IDENTIFY OBSTACLES

You identified obstacles: In the process of preparing your castle, you identified those foods that run counter to your goals, and you identified those obstacles outside the walls of your castle, primarily at work and when eating out. *Phase I/commandment 2*

---

4. CHALLENGE DYSFUNCTIONAL THOUGHTS

You are challenging dysfunctional thoughts relative to your diet and metabolism: ***This is the key***. You understand the truth of a calorie, and that one may not be equivalent to another. You understand the truth of insulin and how that impacts fat metabolism. You understand the truth that obesity is life-limiting. It is the truth about all these things that will help to extinguish the destructive fire that these dysfunctional thoughts are to your health and longevity. *Phase II, III/commandments 5, 8*

---

5. IMPLEMENT BEHAVIORAL ACTIVATION

You are implementing Behavioral Activations, which means that you are modifying your behavior (activation) in the process of achieving your goals, and the positive effects are self-enforcing (20). The very process of reading this manual is activation. Taking the time to read labels, count calories, weigh portion sizes, being honest and being accountable to yourself are all activations.

Implementing an exercise program of even a small but significant amount will provide a sense of accomplishment and well-being. Controlling your calories in, controlling your carbohydrate intake and modulating your insulin levels by fasting are active forms of behavior that will cause positive changes that will begin to correct dysfunctional belief systems relative to nutrition. *Phase II, III, IV/commandments 4, 6, 7, 9, 10*

All the above are logical concrete steps. You check the boxes on the list, and in doing these things you will find success; however, you must not underestimate the power of the Third Arrow, and by that I do not mean only a belief in a higher power, I also mean a belief in yourself, but to believe in yourself, you must know yourself.

As I said at the very beginning, the root cause of obesity is not the food you eat, rather, it is the dysfunctional thoughts you hold in your mind *about* the food you eat. Now, it may be as simple as not being aware of the *Seven Biological Truths* that I have stated, which is easy enough to address. But, what if it's not? What if there is a significant, underlying eating disorder, such as binge eating or a variant thereof?

The incidence of a co-existent eating disorder can be as high as 50% in an obese individual (21). What if there is associated *depression*? An increased incidence of depression is associated with a BMI ≥ 35.

> Obesity can be associated with psychological illnesses, such as depression and eating disorders.

Binge Eating Disorder is associated with *suicidality*, as is the BMI. The BMI has a curvilinear relationship with suicidality, which means that the higher the BMI, the higher the marginal probability of suicidality, and that probability is increased in the presence of a co-existing binge eating disorder (22).

The point I am trying to make is that your needs may be more than can be addressed by a book or manual. In addition, there is some association of psychological pathology, as I referenced above, with the BMI, meaning that the higher your BMI, the higher the probability of a co-existing psychological condition, which can be called a comorbidity. For instance, diabetes, hypertension and coronary heart disease are all comorbidities. Obesity itself is a comorbidity.

Of course, there is no hard number, relative to your BMI, that will be a tell; nor is there an absolute correlation between the BMI and the psychological comorbidities. There will be those with a BMI of less than 35 who suffer depression and those with a BMI greater than 35 who do not; however, I think that the higher your BMI is, the more self-aware you should be that the possibility of dysfunctional thinking runs deeper.

> IF YOU *THINK* YOU SUFFER FROM DEPRESSION OR AN EATING DISORDER, *PLEASE* SEE YOUR PRIMARY CARE PROVIDER FOR ADDITIONAL PROFESIONAL GUIDANCE.

I am talking primarily about the core belief systems that were formed in childhood, belief systems that may have been corrupted by processes you may not even remember. Dysfunctional beliefs lead to negative automatic thoughts and repetitive negative thinking that influence your behavior. Your behavior stimulates a response that can further compound the difficulties of the reality you inhabit. Core beliefs are difficult to change, but they *can be changed*. They must be challenged, and you will change them, but you will need help.

Please recall the brief discussion of Freud's psychoanalytical theory from the arrow of reality section. As always, in the spirit of gross simplification, I see the core beliefs established in childhood as manifestations of the ego and superego, one perched over each shoulder, whispering in your ears the voices only you can hear. *What if they're corrupted*, from whatever process or for whatever reason? What if the voices you hear, your automatic thoughts and assumptions you've drawn from your foundational beliefs, are wrong? What if they are giving faulty advice to your id, your inner baby?

> Your core beliefs need to be healthy. If there is any doubt, seek help.

I have written my manual, *The FAT Thief,* in a specific order because each subsequent phase, arrow and strategy is built on what comes before; and I know that there will be those who won't have to *go all the way* to the terminus of a ketogenic diet with an 18 hour daily fast. It is my intent to harvest the low-hanging fruit as soon as possible, those overweight or obese who don't want to be that way any longer, who do not have severely distorted foundational beliefs or psychological comorbidities. I believe that the self-knowledge gained from knowing the truth will set them free.

But I am esurient. I am using that word because I learned it a few days ago, my *word of the day*, and I liked it. It means *greedy, hungry*. I am esurient for more. I am after the higher-hanging fruit as well. I am after the obese and morbidly obese for whom the promise of a lifelong dietary success has forever been beyond reach.

I believe that if you commit to a belief in yourself--that if you come to know yourself better; that if you can find the serenity to accept the things you cannot change and courage to change the things you can--it is inevitable that hope and success will follow.

If after all this--if after knowing the arrow that be truth; if after knowing the reality of you; if after the contemplation of belief--you struggle still with the slaying of your dragon, there be but three possibilities: The possibility that your foundational beliefs (how you think about yourself) are corrupted: The possibility that the genetic burden of common obesity is a bridge too far for your choice alone to overcome; lastly, the possibility that *it really is a gland problem.*

In the first instance, with professional guidance, courage and faith, you shall overcome. In the second instance, there remains the options of pharmacology and surgical intervention, and you shall overcome. If the final option were to be true, it must first be proved because it is quite rare after all, and if indeed, in the base of your brain, a pituitary tumor does lie, you shall overcome even that, with a craniotomy.

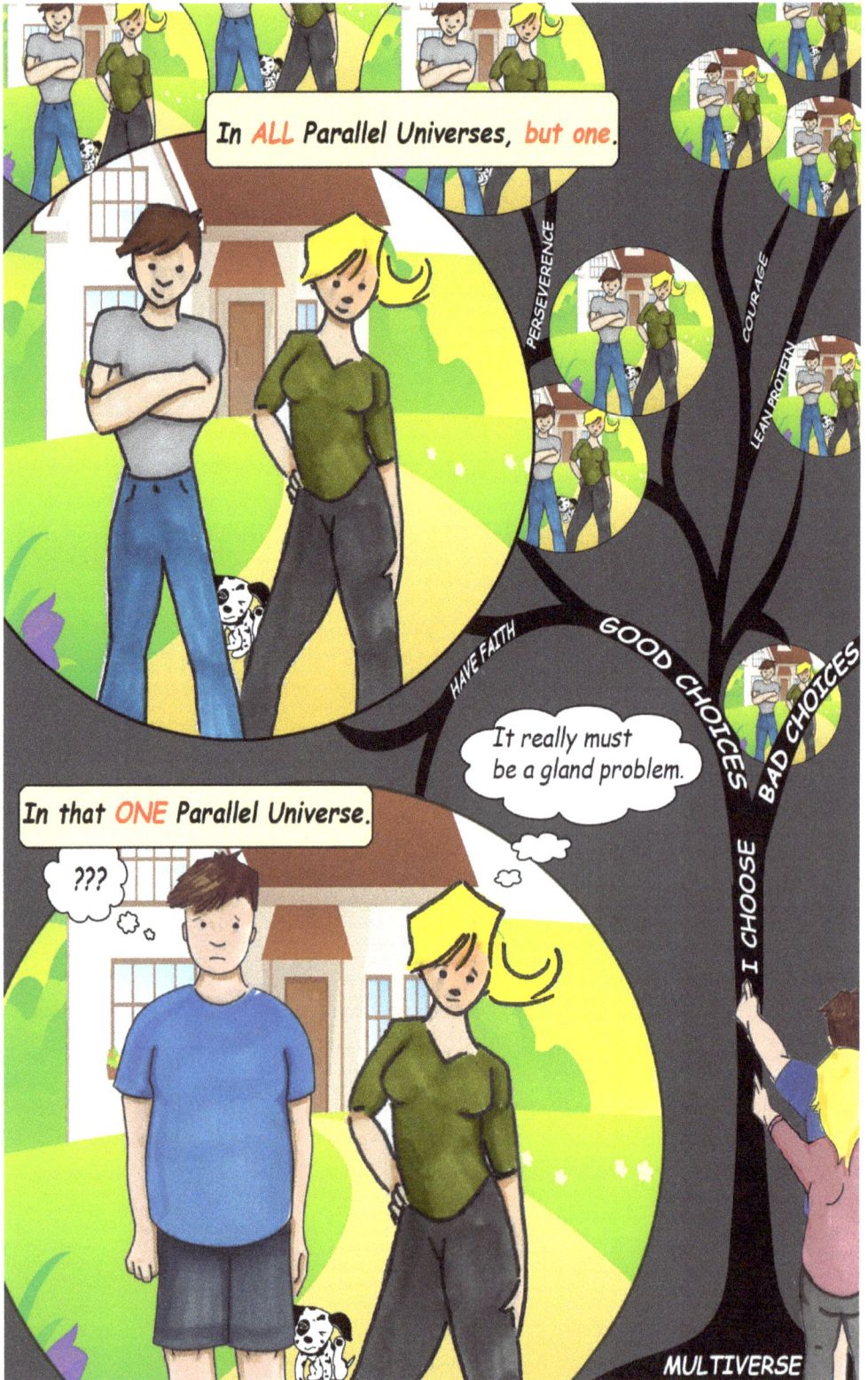

We are almost done, you and I, for now. I have shared everything that I feel to be important as succinctly as I could; however, this thin manual you hold in your hand or in the memory chip of your e-reader is only the beginning. Please think of it as a gateway to a new way of thinking in which you will change your thoughts. There are other books to read, to learn and grow in the process; other people to engage, to friend, to share in the support of a common goal and journey.

Your primary care provider should be involved in your metamorphosis, for that is truly what this will be, in order to manage any comorbidities and medications. There may be a role for professional behavioral management consultation and assistance; however, ultimately, the only thing standing between you and the reality you wish for yourself is *you*. If you can do all these things for yourself; if you can do all these things for those whom you love; if you can do all these things for those who love you; then, you *will change your world.*

What you must do for yourself is most likely not going to be easy. It is going to be hard. It will require patience. It will require perseverance. It will require love and understanding; but, in the end you will come to realize, it is a far far better thing than you have ever done, it is a far far better place than you have ever known.

You need your phone again.

WATCH THE 3RD VIDEO AT FatThief.com

After you read the final chapter, if you choose to do so.

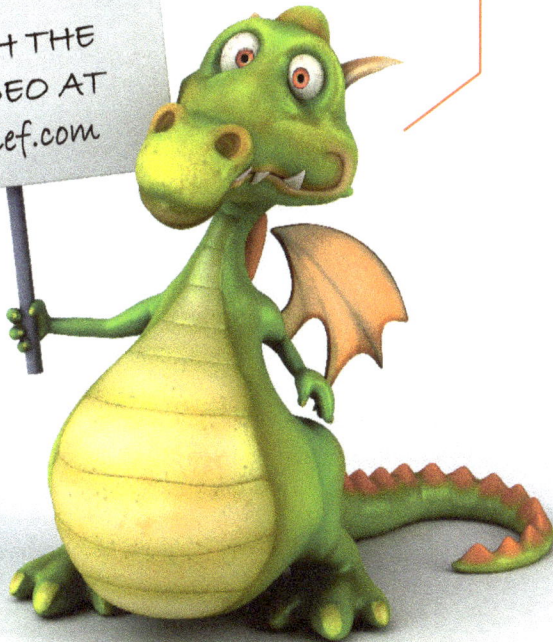

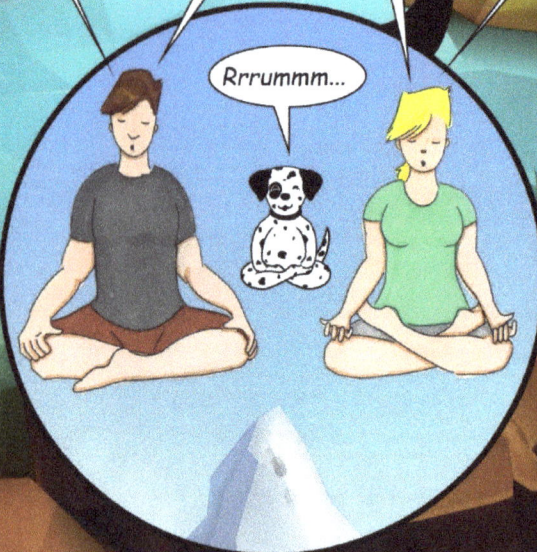

MOMENTS OF GRACE

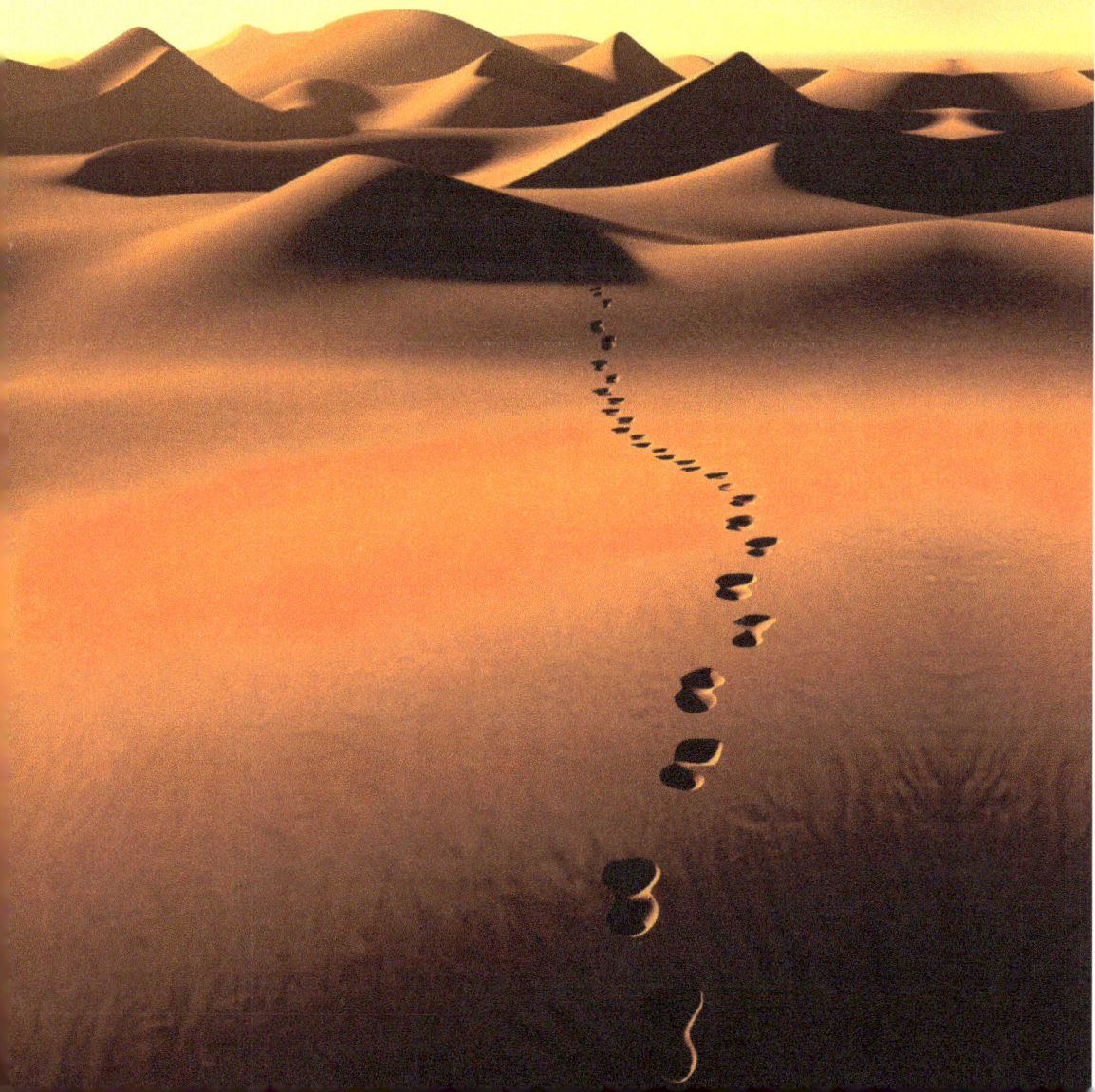

CHAPTER NINE: Belief: Moments of Grace

Clarifications

In my first draft, I led with Faith as the Belief Arrow; however, some of my early readers thought that too exclusive; therefore, I separated Belief into two components; one secular, one spiritual.

I found that I could not completely remove the spiritual from the secular, but I had no difficulty in separating the secular from the spiritual because in manners of spirituality and God, that is really all that matters.

The second component of Belief, your Belief in God as you know Him, will reinforce all that has come before.

Although most of my references are relevant to Christianity and more specifically, Catholicism, that is only because that is what I am most familiar with. It is what works for me. The Eastern religions of Taoism, Hinduism and Buddhism, and the other monotheistic Abrahamic faiths of Judaism and Islam are applicable as well, in accordance to your belief system.

In the process of editing and wrapping things up, I have chosen to rename this final chapter *Moments of Grace*, the reason for which will become clear at the end. We have said goodbye to Dick and Jane and Spot for they have achieved enlightenment, and we need to put any attempt at humor aside for this final chapter, I feel. Now, let's travel back in time several months to the Sunday afternoon when I originally wrote the text of the *Third Arrow of Belief, the First Miracle*.

Something strange happened just now, right this very instant as I was typing this paragraph. I had just finished my story of the miracle that follows and came back to the introduction to insert the clarification that the second component of belief was optional when it happened.

The strange thing that happened was that the music stopped. I was listening to my Pandora station "Enya," which was playing overhead from the Alexa Echo device I had plugged into the receiver in the basement that distributes the signal to all the speakers throughout the house. On the right front corner of my desk, is another Echo device to which I will periodically say, "Alexa, play "____" downstairs," and so she does. I thought I'd try something different but couldn't remember all the selections available on my playlist, so I pulled up the app on my phone to find a different station. The first one I saw, almost like it jumped off the screen was "**Adele** Radio." I don't remember putting it there, but I'm sure I did. I'm listening to it now. You'll see what I mean.

The First Miracle: 1859 (B, 2010)

Those so fortunate as to live here in northeastern Wisconsin, as do I, have the luxury of being quite close to the site of an actual miracle, two miracles really, the site of one of only two Marion Apparitions in the Western hemisphere, so allow me to start there, on the sixth day of October in the year 1859.

It was 11 months to the day before the election of the 16th president of the United States, Abraham Lincoln, and 10 days before John Brown's raid on Harper's Ferry in West Virginia which was a flashpoint for the Civil War. However, in Robinsonville, Wisconsin, October 6th was just another cool day, as most October days are; and the building sounds of war were muted and distant to the ears of 28-year-old **Adele** Brise as she walked along the trail between the trees. The leaves were half-fallen and in various stages of decay on the ground, in the fields and on the paths and roadways. There remained in the branches those more stubborn, not ready to relinquish their spirit until finally pushed off by the abscission cells, the trees telling them, "It is time. It is time." Down, they fell, in twos and threes, slipping and sliding on currents of air, coming to a brief rest only to be rustled across the ground like small animals scurrying. The mornings especially were cool just before dawn, the coolest time of day, and thus it was so on this day as well as Adele walked the four miles from her home in Robinsonville, Wisconsin, to the grist mill halfway between her house and Bay Settlement. In a canvas satchel suspended from a shoulder strap above her right hip she carried a 20-pound bag of wheat to be ground into flour for her family's daily bread. It would weigh slightly less on the return home and would last a week.

The trail was wide enough for two horses abreast, with compacted tracks from the passage of wagons, and Adele walked in the one on the left. She was always told that it was an old Indian trail although she'd never seen an Indian on it; but it was easy for her to imagine lean figures on moccasined feet moving in single file over the soft carpet of dead grass and leaves between the trees.

The shadows of the trees, from the morning sun still low in the Eastern sky, cast the trail in a protracted twilight that would last until late morning, and Adele stepped cautiously over the uneven ground, as one does who has no depth perception, like she has done for most her entire life after becoming blinded in one eye as a young girl. The morning birds singing in the thinned canopy overhead, the crisp sound of her feet pressing into the frosted carpet of leaves, and the earthy smell of composting vegetation peculiar to fall all lent a certain peace to the morning.

Just before the gentle curve in the trail straightened to bring the mill within sight, Adele stopped, startled. Her heart pounded in her chest like it was two sizes too big. She was not alone. There was a lady dressed in white standing in the space between a towering evergreen hemlock and an equally large maple, their branches intersecting overhead at the side of the trail. Adele heard only the sounds of wind-rustled leaves and birdsong overhead. The lady said nothing. She was only a silent presence in the forest, watching her. Adele didn't know what to do. The lady disappeared.

Three days later, on Sunday, October 9th, Adele was walking with her sister, Isabelle, and a neighbor woman, a friend of the family. It was 11 miles on the same trail to the church in Bay Settlement. As they approached that part of the trail before the mill, about half-way to the church, Adele looked towards the space between the maple and hemlock as the three of them drew even with it. Then Adele gasped and suddenly stopped. The other two women saw her standing at the side of the trail, her mouth slightly parted, staring with wide eyes into the emptiness of a space between two trees.

"What's wrong, Adele?" Asked Isabelle.

Adele remained frozen, eyes fixed on the space, silent. She was frightened. She wondered if she'd done something wrong. She searched back in her mind for any memory of a sin inadvertently or openly committed, grave enough to warrant such attention. The lady in white faded to nothing and Adele relaxed, shoulders dropping with a sigh, not knowing quite what to say to her sister and friend.

"Sorry, Isabelle. I thought I saw something."

"What? What did you see?"

"Nothing. Nothing, Isabelle. It was just my imagination. Please, we better go, or we'll be late for church."

After mass, Adele went to confession. She told the priest what had happened to her over the course of the past three days and that she was confused and didn't know what to do. "Have I done something wrong, Father?" she asked.

Father Verhoef had never heard such a tale, but he recalled reading an account of Juan Diego's Marion apparition on the hill of Tepeyac in Mexico written by a seminarian years ago while he himself attended the seminary. Fr. Verhoef was of many years and strong of faith. He said to the girl's shadow from the other side of the porous cloth shade in the small square window of the confessional, "My child, if this lady in white is a heavenly messenger, you will see her again. You must ask her, 'In God's name, who are you and what do you want of me?'"

On the way home that afternoon, at the side of the trail in that same space between the trees the apparition appeared before Adele Brise for the third time. She was the same beautiful woman, clothed in dazzling white, with a yellow sash around her waist. She had a crown of stars around her head.

This time, Adele fell to her knees. "The Lady," she gasped, then she asked the question Father had suggested, "In God's name, who are you and what do you want of me?"

The Lady lifted her hands as though she were to embrace Adele and said, "I am the Queen of Heaven, who prays for the conversion of sinners, and I wish you to do the same. You received the Holy Communion this morning, and that is well. But you must do more..."

The other two women saw Adele kneeling in the grass before the space in the trees. "Adele, who is it?" asked her sister.

"Why can't we see her as you do?" asked the neighbor-lady who was frightened and began crying.

"Kneel," said Adele, "the Lady says she is the Queen of Heaven."

They both knelt, tears running down their cheeks. The Queen of Heaven turned to them and said, "Blessed are they that believe without seeing..." but they heard nothing other than the soft rustle of wind through the branches and leaves falling.

"What more can I do, dear Lady?" asked Adele, the vision bright and shiny through a film of tears.

"Gather the children in this wild country, and teach them what they should know for salvation."

"But how shall I teach them who know so little myself?"

"Teach them," the Queen of Heaven told her, "teach them their catechism, how to make the Sign of the Cross, and how to approach the sacraments; that is what I wish you to do. Go now, and fear nothing. I will help you." She lifted her hand as though giving a blessing and was gone.

It was Sunday, October 9th, 1859.

Teach the children the Lady in white told Marie Adele Joseph Brise. And so, she did.

The Second Miracle: 1871

Over the course of the ensuing 12 years, the Civil War came, and the Civil War went. Across America's fruited plains, wave after wave of gray had crashed against wave after wave of blue, each spending itself on the other amid the sounds of muskets and cannon and the cries of rage and pain emblematic of man's inhumanity to man. Slowly, a nation healed; and, in northeast Wisconsin, Adele worked on her mission. Her father, Lambert, built a chapel on the grounds of where the Queen of Heaven appeared to her. In 1864 a school and convent were built, and in 1869 the chapel school was opened. It was named St. Mary's Boarding Academy.

Which brings us to the fall of 1871, the month of October once again, except that this year the weather was unseasonably warm and dry with below average precipitation in the months of June, July, August and September. Small fires smoldered in the fields as the lands were cleared after the harvest in preparation for the following year's planting. In the early afternoon of October 8th, the wind picked up out of the south and west as a low-pressure system from the warm air rising into the atmosphere moved over southwestern Minnesota. It ran up against a high-pressure system centered on Virginia and the Carolinas. The two systems of drastically different temperatures and humidity sought equilibrium. By 2 p.m. the wind was steady at 10-15 mph, with gusts up to 20-30 mph.

Remember, it was Sunday. Families were preparing meals at home. Church was done. Adele was preparing for the following week's lessons at the school; and just south of New Franken a small pile of brush gently glowed, sending a thin trail of smoke heavenward, a signal, except that there were none to receive it. A gust of wind roiled over the ground and embers, smoldering red, became instantly a rain of fire.

The fires coalesced into a wall of flames hundreds of feet high that raced over the tinder-dry fields of cornstalks, mown hay and harvested wheat. The flames leapt from the fields to the trees, engulfing the canopies of dried residual leaves. The trees burned from the top down; pillars of fire so closely spaced as to become one. The firestorm was a self-propagating monster of death with whirlwinds of tornadic destruction over 1,000 meters in height and horizontal roll vortices with winds well in excess of 100 mph, strong enough to uproot the trees as they burned. The fire advanced North and East on both sides of the Bay of Green Bay faster than man or animal could run.

Families and communities in its path were powerless. The sound of the fire was as the roar of a jet engine on the ground approaching. An intense, dry heat preceded the flames that only accentuated the terror of the death coming. Inside the fire, the temperatures exceeded 2,000 degrees Fahrenheit. The surface of the sun is 10,000 degrees. It's as though the sun reached out with a long, thin finger of flame of almost sentient precision, so focal was its caress.

The people of Robinsonville had no place to go. The wall of flame and wind from the South wouldn't allow the time necessary to move to the lake; so, instead, they took their families and livestock into the church yard, five acres of grass and buildings demarcated by a white wooden fence of sections of horizontal bars within which stood a church, its sharp steeple piercing the sky, a sky filling with heat and smoke.

The families gathered the elderly and children in the church while outside Sister Adele prayed the Rosary, holding a statue of the Blessed Mother high as she marched around the yard, the able-bodied men and women of Robinsonville following behind, praying for mercy and salvation. With cloths over their faces to filter the smoke and ash, they prayed. With the arid, intense heat drying the tears on their faces, they prayed. Inside the flames that burned and raged at close of day, they prayed in unison. "Hail Mary, full of Grace...", they said over and over as animals of the wild, small and large, crept under the fence and through the gates into the churchyard as all night long the fires burned.

In the darkness of early morning, rain begin to fall, and when the morning's cool light came to the eyes of the people of Robinsonville, they saw the blackness and destruction surrounding them on all sides, stretching to the horizons; North South East and West. The ash and cinder reached up to the charred outer surfaces of a wooden fence that on the inside was yet still white, a fence that surrounded an untouched oasis of green, within which stood a church with a sharp steeple piercing the sky, and in and about the church, all the people. It's as though God himself reached out from Heaven with a finger of grace to touch the face of the Earth, as if to say, "Not here. Not here."

It was the morning of October 9th, in that place, where 12 years earlier, to the day, the Queen of Heaven visited Marie Adele Joseph Brise. Upwards of 2,500 people had perished. Towns disappeared from the map. The Earth was a black and smoldering ruin along both sides of the bay but for that one small circle of green, like a sparkling emerald dropped from the sky.

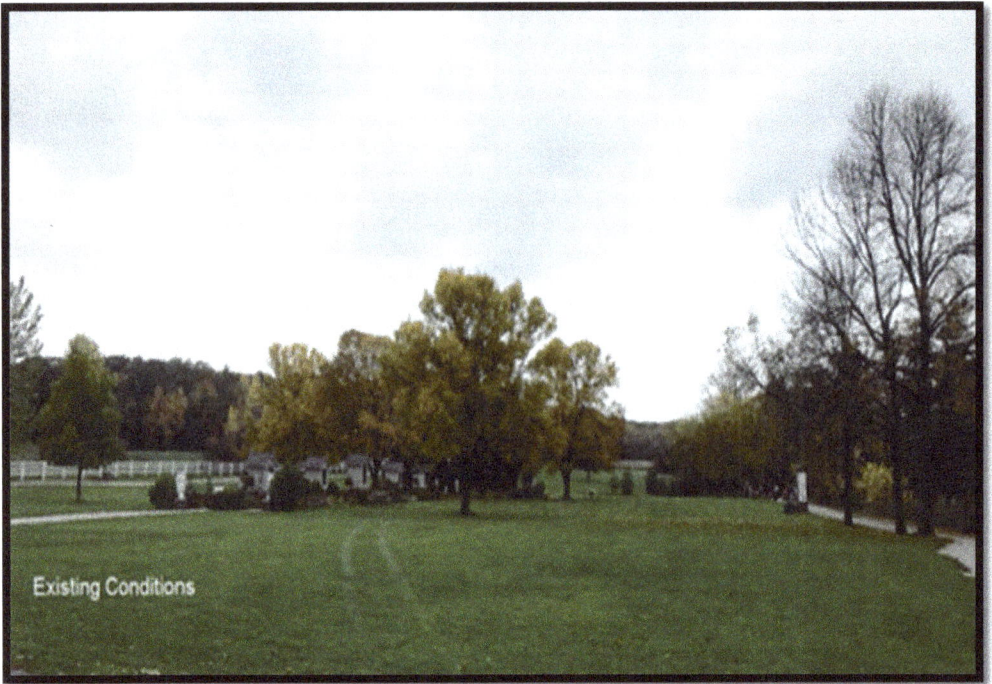

Existing Conditions

The current day grounds of the site of the first two miracles in Champion, WI. You can see the white fence demarcating the Church grounds.

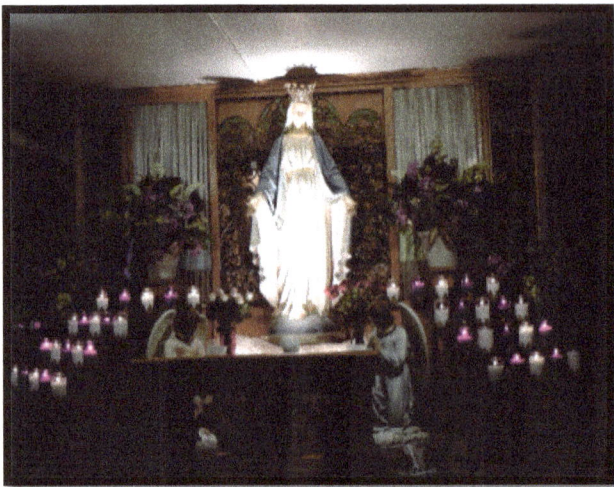

The National Shrine of
Our Lady of Good Help
Champion, WI.

Part III: The Third Miracle: 1966

Had it been raining, nothing bad would have happened because she would have stayed inside. But the sun was out, three quarters advanced across the early evening sky, and the gentle breeze, warm and humid from the South, was more suggestive of a full summer day than the early spring it was. Half a world away, young men; husbands, sons, brothers, but mostly sons and brothers were stepping off troop transport planes into the fetid, oppressive heat of Operation Rolling Thunder. By the end of that year of 1966 the number of U.S. forces in Vietnam would have climbed to 385,000. However, in early May, it remained something mostly in the news and on the college campuses except for the thousands of families so directly afflicted. It was certainly not on the young woman's mind as she left the apartment building in Moorhead, Minnesota, a square-ish dirty brown brick six-plex where she lived in a modest unit on the second floor with her husband and two children.

They had picked the Miller apartments for its location, facing a quiet side street, an elementary school with a playground down the block on the corner. It was the playground that she took her children to in the mornings, and sometimes in the evenings after dinner, as was the case this evening. Her husband was in the apartment getting ready to cover a school board meeting for the local radio station. The young woman crossed the small grass boulevard, holding her 2-year-old girl in her left arm, grasping the small hand of her 4-year-old boy in her right. She stopped before the curb of the southern side of 19th St. South, a not quite through street intersecting 9th Avenue that ran East and West. Their apartment complex of three buildings was in the southwest corner of the intersection. On the northern side of 19th street lay the three-city-block rectangle of Romkey Park, and a playground.

There was no car in sight. It was almost quiet. The soft background noise of a lawn mower from the house to the East of the apartment complex mixed with the songs of robins and the sound of budding branches rustling together in the gentle wind that carried the scent of rain not far off. The children were already excited, especially the oldest, who was at that age where he could do things over and over and over again and derive just as much enjoyment with the last occurrence as with the first. She looked both ways, then looked down at her son, smiling, "Do you see any cars?" She asked, knowing already the answer.

"No, Mommy."

"OK then; look both ways," she said, demonstrating with exaggerated turns of her head, like she did every time. Then, holding her daughter in her left arm, she stepped into the street, the boy at her side, holding his left hand in her right. They crossed safely. In the distance, from the North, another engine, like a lawn mower, but not, went unnoticed.

From the apartment-side of the street from which they had just left a young voice rings out, "Hi," excited as only an almost 4-year-old could be at seeing a familiar figure. He cries out again, "Hi," a tiny arm raised. It is the other boy's best friend from a unit on the third and highest level of the same building. The friend's unit was the exact mirror opposite of his own, which they collectively found strangely fascinating, as well as the relative height of a third-story window and the particular effect that that had on delicate objects dropped through a not quite accidental rent in the window screen.

"It's Tony, Mommy."

The boy pulls away and turns back to the street, but he is already 4 and so he knows not to step into the street, he only stands on the curb. He raises his hand and waves back and forth with fingers spread, a wide smile at being recognized, feeling important for it. "Hi, Tony," he yells back across the street. That is all he remembers. His mother screams.

A 19-year-old man was looking for an address on an unfamiliar street. He was picking up a girl from his Art History class that he had finally hit it off with before the end of the term. They were going to a protest on the campus. All of his friends were against the war in Vietnam, and somebody famous, a woman, was giving a talk in the Union square. He couldn't remember who it was exactly, but someone who had been on TV or in a movie or at least was going to be in a movie. It was going to be a great time.

He couldn't remember if it was 1001, or 801, but he knew that she drove a powder blue VW Beetle with peace signs on the doors, a *Make Love, Not War* sticker on the front hood and a *Give Peace a Chance* sticker on the back. He couldn't wait to give peace a chance. The rumble of his bike transfused his body like he was a part of it, or it a part of him. He wore a red bandana and a sleeveless jean jacket with a peace sign on the back. His brown hair waved behind him like a torn flag in the wind. He saw a number…1002; on the west side of the street, on his right. Damn. Did I miss it, he thought?

He gripped the handlebars firmly and quickly looked over his right shoulder to see if there was a dirty blue egg-shape on the side of the road. He didn't even see the boy as his bike crossed into the oncoming lane. He heard a woman scream and reflexively released the throttle and squeezed the brake levers, but not before feeling the impact of a small body against his left handle-bar; but what he found most distressing was the crisp sound of the impact, like the head of a hammer against the yielding surface of an un-ripened melon.

She thought he was safe. She was already across the street with her children, but she was a worrier, and the snarl of the engine approaching made her nervous. Clutching her girl tightly, she reached out to pull her son back. Then she saw the motor bike swerve towards her side of the street. She was so close, her fingertips on the fabric of his shirt. She heard a woman screaming, not recognizing the sound of her own voice. Then, just like that, he was gone; picked up by the handlebar of the motor bike; a handlebar that stood at the precise height of a male, 4-years-old, height in the 90th percentile. The force of the impact drove the bar into the delicate shell of the boy's right temporal parietal skull, rupturing the protective overlying dura, driving sharp fragments of bone deep into the sacred tissues of action and thought. The small body was picked up, as if by a hand, and carried 50 feet along the pavement before the inertia of forward movement overcame the deceleration of the bike.

The boy spun around 360 degrees, his right arm still held aloft, as though in a pirouette, before dropping to the pavement with a soft thud, landing on his back. His head bounced once, then a second time, gentler, before coming to a rest, turned sharply to his left, devoid of all muscular tone. From the crushed inward depression in the right side of his skull, blood welled up like a shallow cup of thick red wine overflowing. His mother ran towards him, arms outstretched, mouth opened wide. The primeval scream that escaped from the fracture in her soul shattered the evening quiet, silencing the birds overhead such that the cries of the mother and young man in the street that came after were magnified, a cacophony of despair, the sound of death, nearby. In the street her son waited, eyes open but unseeing, a red halo expanding.

In the emergency room, minutes later, the boy was non-responsive, but breathing. Dr. Lee Christoferson, the neurosurgeon on call that evening stated in the medical record:

"Upon my arrival, the child's pupils were equal and reactive to light, his eyes were divergent, however. He seemed to have a positive left Babinski. Abdominal reflexes were absent."

A positive Babinski is an abnormal response to a normal reflex obtained when the lateral aspect of the sole of the foot is stroked. The normal response is for the toes to curl downward. The abnormal response is for the big toe to curl up, which suggests a spinal cord injury or other severe central nervous system pathology.

Dr Christoferson then further stated in the medical record:

"On reviewing the x-rays, he had an area which appeared to be approximately 6cm in diameter and rather rounded that was markedly depressed, being depressed in the brain what I estimated to be about 4 cm."

The CT scan was invented in 1972, eight years subsequent in Dr. Christoferson's career; therefore, the x-rays he refers to are plain films demonstrating only the bony elements of the skull. Films that are now merely of historical interest, darkly translucent, silver-impregnated sheets hung on light boxes in which the white shadows of bones are seen against the exposed, light-blackened silver where the bones are not.

Minutes before Dr. Christoferson took the boy to surgery, after being emergently transported to the tertiary care center where he worked, he documented:

"I carried out a brief re-check. At this time his right pupil is dilated as compared with the left."

The operative report of Dr. Lee Christoferson, 17 May 1966:

Pre-operative Diagnosis: *Depressed skull fracture right parietal.*
Post-operative Diagnosis: *Same with severe cerebral laceration, laceration of posterior branch of the middle cerebral artery and severe intracerebral hematoma.*
Operation: *Elevation and excision of depressed skull fracture. Evacuation of intracerebral hemorrhage with ligation of bleeding artery.*

Procedure: *... the child was turned slightly on his left side and the scalp of the right side of the head was shaved and was then prepared and draped in the usual manner. A horseshoe shaped incision was made beginning above the ear*
.... out from beneath the scalp, bubbled out a large amount of degenerated necrotic brain tissue with blood clot.
...From the central area of the depressed area of skull was a rather active bleeder and coming up from the depressed central area was a considerable amount of necrotic brain.
...and then I was able to lift up and remove the two depressed fragmented pieces of bone inferiorly.
... was an enormous amount of blood clot and bleeding occurring. I lifted up the dura here and began to evacuate clot from his brain and a total of clot measuring almost the size of a tennis ball...
...The laceration of the brain was retracted and in the depths was found a very large branch of the middle cerebral artery...
...until all bleeding points had been coagulated and the brain was perfectly dry.

In the waiting area outside the operating suite, the boy's mother softly cried, kneeling on the floor, her head cradled on clasped hands resting on the seat of a chair. It was after midnight, the room was empty but for her murmur of urgently repeated Hail Mary's between sobs, the ritualistic prayer forming a protective barrier between the memory of her little angel in the street and her sanity. She refused to leave the one space in the universe that was the absolute closest she could physically be to her son. In the hospital chapel at the far end of the hall, the boy's father prayed. He gave his son up to God. His head slumped forward as the tension left with the breath in his body. Then, like a light illuminating the darkness, he knew that his son would live.

He raced back to the waiting area to tell his wife that their child would be okay and, in the hallway, leading from the operating room he ran into Dr. Christoferson.

"How is my son?" he asked.

"Your son is alive. He will live, but there is a high likelihood that he will be paralyzed on the left side of his body; but I did my job. My job was to save his life."

"Thank you, doctor," the father said in a tremulous whisper.

"Don't thank me. Thank God," said Dr. Christoferson, looking into the father's eyes, his focus fading into infinity. The timbre of his voice dropped an octave it seemed as he continued, "When I ligated the bleeding artery deep inside the brain, one of the main arteries to that part of the brain, all the bleeding stopped, and I saw the other blood vessels fill and grow before my eyes. I have never seen that before."

"It was a miracle," he said.

19 May 1966

The little boy was two days removed from his accident, sedated, but breathing on his own. His scalp had been closed over the silver-dollar sized hole in the skull, a soft spot, like the fontanelles a baby is born with. The swollen brain pushed up against it, a hole without which the intracranial pressure would have been too great. In the bed next to the boy was another boy, one year older, who had been kicked in the head by a horse. It was his second week in a coma. The respective mothers didn't know each other, separated by a curtain, each in permanent residence on the far sides of the beds, relative to each other, each immersed in the tragedy their lives had become.

Dr. Christoferson walked into the room, tall, thin, severe. He said good morning to the mother and father, then examined his patient, listening to his heart and lungs, eliciting bilateral patellar reflexes, checking for a Babinski sign. He lifted his head and looked across the bed at the parents, "I think it's time we let him wake up. Remember," he continued, "although I have not been able to elicit evidence of paralysis yet, he sustained a severe brain injury and likely will not have the full use of the left side of his body."

Two hours later, after lunch, the boy's father slipped a new pair of tennis shoes on his son's feet and asked him if he remembered how to tie his shoes like he was taught the week before the accident. The boy bent up his left leg and with both hands, crossed one large loop over the other and completed the tie. His parents cried.

————————————

More than 40 years passed. The CT scan, which was invented in 1972, became nearly as common as a CXR. In 1989, the boy graduated from medical school, and in 1994 from a surgery program. In 1997 the Green Bay Packers won Super Bowl XXXI. In 2006 the boy, who had become a surgeon himself, lost his mind for 12 hours, which turned out to be of no great consequence as the ultimate cause proved to be that of sleep-deprivation from being on-call 10 days in a row; however, in 2006, such a gap in memory triggered many tests, one of the first being a brain CT scan, his first. Ever. Shortly after he returned to the emergency room from the radiological suite, the reading radiologist, working from an offsite facility, called the ER physician who had evaluated the boy who became a man who became a surgeon. He asked, "Can this man walk?"

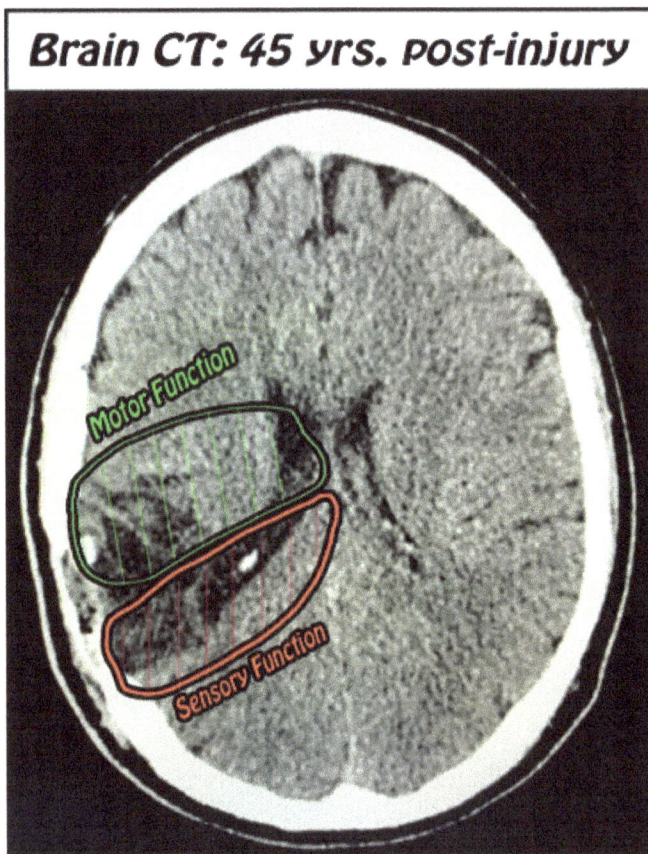

Brain CT: 45 yrs. post-injury

Miracle: (noun): a surprising and welcome event that is not explicable by natural scientific laws and is therefore considered to be the work of a divine agency. "His first miracle was to turn water into wine."

Dictionary.com

So. A miracle requires a belief in let's just say, God, as opposed to a "higher power." I've told you a true story, mildly fictionalized, based on historical records and the writing of *Fr. Edward Looney* of the Green Bay Diocese (23). I've also told you a true story based on factual medical records and personal interviews of the involved persons dealing with a traumatic brain injury. I don't expect that I'll make a true believer from telling a few stories. My purpose in telling you these stories is simply to present an argument for the reality of miracles, or at least the reality of belief, over and above all the other miracles we grew up with, like the parting of the Red Sea; the turning of water into wine at Cana, you saved the best wine for last; the rising of Lazarus, and all the other biblical miracles you learned over the years.

All these miracles, recently referenced, are big miracles, grand miracles that would likely give even a doubting Thomas pause; but, what about all the smaller ones that fill our lives on almost a daily basis. What about the time you stepped on the gas to make a left turn onto a busy highway, then looked one more time to your right and saw an approaching vehicle, and stepped on the brake instead? How about when someone you knew, or a loved one, or even you yourself received a diagnosis of cancer, and survived? What about the time you were driving down a street and a voice tells you to slow down or stop, and a small child runs out from behind a parked car? Everyone has experiences like these. Everyone.

So, you believe in God. You believe in a higher power. How does that become an arrow?

If you believe in miracles, or at least your heart is open to a belief in miracles, that means that you recognize the reality of divine intervention. That means that the God-arrow is yours. And that means, like a mythical King Arthur pulling the sword from stone, you are worthy to pull the God-arrow from the imaginary quiver on your back. You are worthy.

The problem with the God-arrow is that you only think to use it for the big things, like if you think you're going to die. The answer is that you must learn to use it with the little things too. It's not like He's only there for the big things. He's there for everything. Every. Little. Thing.

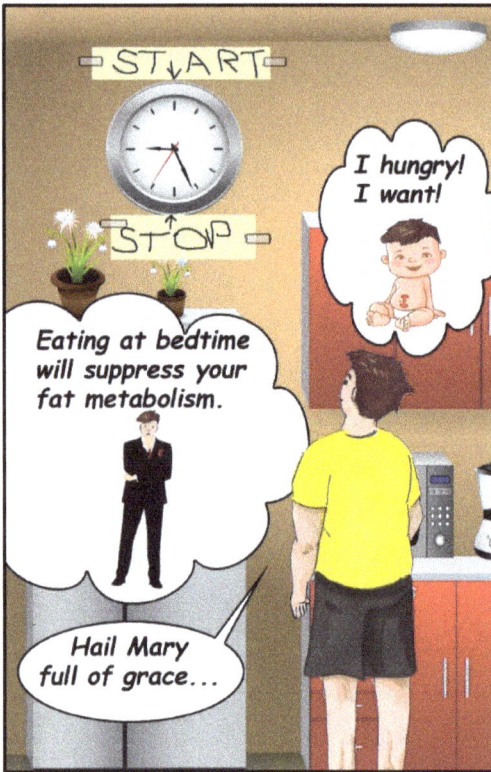

It's not like *Oh, my God. I'm going to die, please save me* is the only time you think you can use the God-arrow, like when you're lying on your back in a PET scanner at the Mayo Clinic listening to a mother sing a lullaby to her young child with cancer behind the closed curtained cubicle against the wall opposite, and it's so sad you find yourself quietly crying.

No, that's not it at all. You can use the God-Arrow for every day, for everything that is important to you, which, in this case, specifically, is for maintaining the health and purity of the temple of your spirit that is your physical body.

How do you do this? How do you use the God-arrow for weight-loss?

I am not suggesting that you go full St. Francis and give away all your worldly possessions to live a life of poverty, chastity and start a leper colony on some remote island or compound in the Northwoods. I'm not even suggesting that you go to church or pray every day, although any combination of the above would likely be a net positive in the hereafter. I am merely suggesting that you access your faith in your higher power to help you in all those little decisions you make throughout each and every day, all those choices that lead directly to the self-deterministic reality you find yourself within.

It is difficult for anyone to imagine themselves as a saint. I doubt that even Sister Theresa imagined herself as a saint, but one day she started, and, well, one thing led to another. But *she started*. That's the take-home message.

I am also not suggesting that I am an expert in the prayerful aspects of your life. I am an expert in things medical and metabolic, but not in this. I am not part of the clergy. Your belief in the Divine is a deeply personal part of your life, and it is not my position to lend council other than my own personal feelings and what I have found helpful. The are no limits to your own application of the Divine to your recovery and are only dependent on your own God-given imagination, wisdom and religious counsel.

So, now that I've established my role in this second component of the Belief Arrow; and apart from becoming a saint in your imitation of Christ, or at least *starting to become*, how might you use your faith in the little ways to guide you in your small daily sacrifices in making choices and choosing well?

Below is a list of strategies that I have found helpful personally. Perhaps you will find them helpful as well. As with all my lists of suggestions, there are no limits, they are not complete, there are additional strategies you will find and employ that are specific to you, and *Blessings to You* in that regard.

List of Strategies using Faith for the little things.

---

1.   *Begin each day with a prayer.*

Begin each day with a prayer specific to your goal. This could be on first awaking, or if you're rushed, while brushing your teeth, or in the shower. It could be formulaic prayer or simply your own words asking Him for strength, for compassion, for patience, for skill, for whatever it is you think you need that day.

Some may find it helpful to have a daily meditation or prayer book with a special reflection for each new day.

---

2.   *End each day in a similar way.*

End each day a similar way, with a prayer, the last thing. *Now I lay me down to sleep…*

Reflect on what you did well, what you could have done better, what you would have done differently.

---

3. When you are presented with a choice for which you know the right answer but are struggling with, say a prayer.

We constantly find ourselves in the position of wanting to do something, the easier choice, the path of least resistance, following the way of the pleasure principle; and you know there is a better way, the moral way, the WWJD way. So, stop. Say a prayer. *WWJD=What would Jesus Do?*

This could be a short formulaic prayer such as the Serenity Prayer or a Hail Mary. This does two things: It allows time to think, time for your better selves, the ego and superego to rev up and provide the id with reason and rationale to not do what you really want to do but know you shouldn't. The second thing it does is provide at least a small portion of God's Grace for the moment, that transient little burst of resolve that just might be enough.

---

4. Use a religious talisman

Use a religious talisman as a reminder of your commitment to God, and to yourself. I have several. I wear a Christian wedding ring and a Jerusalem Cross always; both blessed, both having touched the birthplace of Jesus.

At work I have a medallion hanging on a hook in the back of my locker along with a 5 x7 in. glass-covered picture of Jesus, holding his hand up in benediction, from the year 1953. It's a small calendar. My grandfather used to give them out to customers of his small grocery store on South 10th St. in Bismarck, ND during the depression years. A talisman can be felt, it can be seen, it can be a reminder and a source of strength for you.

---

5. Use a religious Mantra

These are short and immediate; they may be the first thing you do when presented with a choice. They may be repeated throughout the day during a quiet time or during a stressful time. A few Christian mantras would be *Jesus, pray for me; For Thine is the Kingdom and the power and the glory; I am that I am.*

---

6. Display reminders of your faith and commitment.

Display reminders of your faith and commitment where you need them most. I already mentioned my locker at work. It is a source of comfort for me, a place of reflection. I also have a second picture of Jesus from Grandpa's store perched on top of a thick-framed picture of Einstein that hangs opposite the desk in my office. In my office at home I have a small olivo-wood statue of Jesus holding a Roman guard with a hammer. The statue is called, "Forgiven."

You could hang a religious medal or icon in the kitchen, inside the door of a cupboard, on the side of the fridge. These present emotional, Godly reminders to you. I suppose that a Rosary looped through the handles of the fridge would be an example of a mechanical barrier; but that would quickly become tiresome, I fear.

---

7. Once a week, do something bigger

Once a week, do something bigger. For me, this is going to church. It takes an hour. I am more or less alone with my thoughts. You can't talk. It is a special place and a special time. For others, this could be a different special place; a place that is quiet and free from distraction and conducive to deep thoughts and reflection. This time, once a week, is a removal from the earthly world and the constant noise that is in your head and all around.

I am going to stop with the list of the little things now, not because I am done, but because I must stop somewhere, and this place seems as good as any, and I like the number seven. Like I said, it's lucky; and, on the seventh day, He rested.

I am going to end now. Other than editing and corrections, this is the last thing I will write for my manual for you. It is all done, after this. I did not have this before this morning. Interestingly, as with my last effort 10 years ago with the *Relativity Diet,* a much larger and rarely read book, the ending came to me in church.

THE FINAL WORD, FINALLY

The last time I wrote a book, the ending came to me in church on a Sunday morning in the summer. It came from Proverbs, 8:27-31. I can't remember if it was the first or second reading, but when I heard it, I knew that was how I wanted to end it. *This is it*, I whispered to myself.

This time, the ending came to me on a Sunday morning in the fall. It came from the Homily, which was drawn from the readings. I don't think I would have arrived at it without the sermon; therefore, I must thank *Fr. Ryan Krueger of Corpus Christi* in Sturgeon Bay, WI, for his sermon on that day.

In my list of seven little things, what all of them depend upon is a moment of Grace, a brief moment of strength from God who is within you and with you always; a transient resolve to do the thing you'd rather not, to make the right choice, the Godly choice. It is appropriate to now end with the biggest thing.

In his sermon, Fr. Krueger presented two extreme examples of moments of Grace and then made the similar point, as I did in the list above, that moments of Grace don't have to be extreme or momentous or infrequent. They are daily, for He is always with you, there for you, whenever you ask or call or need.

The extreme examples of moments of Grace Fr. Ryan discussed dealt with the supreme sacrifice, the sacrifice of self. If you recall, I discussed the role of sacrifice and self-denial in the first component of the Arrow of Belief, but the discussion was not complete for the reason that the ultimate sacrifice would be the sacrifice of life, to give one's life for a larger purpose, and I believe that requires a belief in God, or if you prefer, a belief in a power greater than self.

Consider the Christian martyrs: the first martyr, St. Stephan, stoned to death by the Sanhedrin for preaching against the temple; or St. Paul who was beheaded by Nero at the Aquae Salviae in Rome; or St. Peter who was crucified upside down by the same. And of course, there remains the most supreme sacrifice of all: *For God so loved the world that he gave his one and only son.* This was illustrated in a most beautiful and poignant way in Mel Gibson's *The Passion of Christ.* I can still see the images of Jim Caviezel, as Jesus, being scourged, skin shredded, bleeding, the crown of thorns, dying on the cross, and thinking *it must have been exactly like that.*

In today's sermon by Fr. Ryan, his first extreme example of a moment of Grace dealt with St. Paul, but before getting to that, I wanted to share with you my thoughts of St. Paul I had earlier this year during a pilgrimage to the Holy Land. It was March 16th of 2019, a beautiful day on the southeastern slope of

Mount Hermon in Israel, looking down on Syria and the road to Damascus. The exact place of the conversion of St. Paul was demarcated by a faintly seen church steeple, close to a more readily seen airport tower that the guide initially drew our attention to.

Obviously, there wasn't a physical road in our time, but I could imagine the road that St. Paul traveled on the day of his conversion. I think that St. Paul is as about as much proof of God as anything else you might encounter other than your own conversion or miracle. Thing is, St. Paul never met Jesus. Imagine that. Not only that, but he killed Christians at the time. He was present at the stoning of St. Stephan, the first Christian martyr, outside the Lion's Gate of Jerusalem; probably gave the order; and, on the day of his conversion he was traveling to Damascus to pick up a group of the new Christian sect to bring back to Jerusalem for persecution.

Imagine that. Imagine a homely Roman Pharisee, known as Saul of Tarsus, historically described as a short, bald-headed, bow-legged man with a large nose, trotting along on his horse on the road to Damascus, lost in his thoughts of new ways to persecute followers of that problematic Jewish false-prophet called Jesus; followers, followers everywhere, sprouting up like weeds from cracks in the earth after a rain.

Imagine Saul coming to that spot within sight of the walls of Damascus where he was suddenly blinded by a light so bright that it took his sight; then, from the heavens overhead, a voice, "Saul, Saul, why do you persecute me?"

Imagine Saul being led by his traveling companions, who did not hear the voice or see the light, the rest of the way to Damascus. Imagine the state Saul must have been in. He remained in the city for three days in a house on the Via Recta, praying, when on the third day a man called Ananias, sent by God, placed his hands over Saul's eyes and restored his sight.

Saul was baptized by Ananias, changed his name to Paul, spent the next 30 years being chased, imprisoned, persecuted, and finally executed for his belief in Jesus as the Son of God; and all the while writing, teaching, and becoming the most influential Christian in the promulgation of a faith that spread across world over the course of the subsequent 2,000 years. That is a brief history of St. Paul.

How could that possibly happen if it wasn't true? There are really only two possibilities: either Saul of Tarsus was a genius paranoid schizophrenic with delusions of grandeur who *thought* he heard the voice of God, and was so convinced that he spent the next 30 years responding to that delusion, changing the very course of humankind and suffering all the while; or, St. Paul *did hear* the voice of God, after which everything else becomes rational and believable as by far the simplest explanation and thereby most likely to be the correct one in accordance with Occam's razor. The final emphasis of St. Paul's faith is found at his end of his days, as demonstrated by his letter to Timothy, 4:6-8, 16-18, written the night before his beheading by Nero in Rome. This night before his death was Fr. Ryan's first extreme example of moments of Grace.

St. Paul wrote:

I am already being poured out as a libation and **the time of my departure has come**. I have fought the good fight, I have finished the race, I have kept the faith. From now on there is reserved for me the crown of righteousness, which the Lord, the righteous judge, will give me on that day and not only to me but also to all who have longed for his appearing.

At my first defense no one came to my support, but all deserted me. **May it not be counted against them!** But **the Lord stood by me and gave me strength**, so that through me the message might be fully proclaimed and all the Gentiles might hear it. So I was rescued from the lion's mouth. The Lord will rescue me from every evil attack and save me for his heavenly kingdom. To him be the glory forever and ever. Amen. *(emphasis mine)*

In Paul's letter to Timothy, who was as a son to him, he writes that he knows he's going to die, that he is at peace with that, and that he forgives those who were not there when he needed them. He writes of how God was always there for him in those dark hours when he needed Him most.

His letter to Timothy, the night before his death, is only one moment of Grace he had experienced in his 30-year ministry, a moment of Grace at the end of his life that gave him the peace and strength to forgive those who abandoned him and to accept his death for the Heavenly Kingdom.

Fr. Ryan's second example was Saint Maximilian Kolbe, a Catholic priest imprisoned in Auschwitz during WWII. In his second month of imprisonment, 10 men were randomly chosen from a line-up for execution by starvation and dehydration. He was not chosen, but when one of the 10 began pleading for mercy because he had a wife and children Fr. Kolbe stepped forward and told the guards to take him, "I would like to take that man's place. He has a wife and children."

Fr. Kolbe and the nine others were locked in a below ground room where they sang hymns and prayed for the next two weeks until Fr. Kolbe and three others were the last ones remaining. The guards, who had been hearing hymns and prayers wafting up through the grates all the while, could stand it no longer. They put him and the others to death by lethal injection. Fr. Maximilian reportedly held out his arm for the needle, then raised his arm while the drug ran in. (24)

These burdens born by St. Paul and St. Maximilian seem impossible to me from the outside looking in, much as the burdens born by family members and friends dealing with the loss of a spouse, or the loss of a child, the diagnosis of a terminal illness. The pain, the loss, the emptiness in the fabric of them, the approach of an earthly death decades too early seems unimaginable to me. How do they do it? I don't know if I could bear it. *How could I?*

Moments of Grace. I believe that our lives are a succession of moments of Grace, much of the time unaware of His presence supporting us, lifting us up; those times in our life when there is only one set of footsteps in the sand because we are being carried by our Lord. There will be small moments and there will be large moments, and all you must do is believe and know that He will be there.

In the picture of Fr. Maximilian Kolbe, you see an austere, perhaps stern, man, much like any other. It is not too difficult to imagine him fasting or suffering for his belief, but if you saw his picture *not in the context of his story* you would not know him capable of such a sacrifice as he made. It is possible, even likely, that he did not know himself until that moment--that moment of Grace, when he stepped forward and said, "Take me."

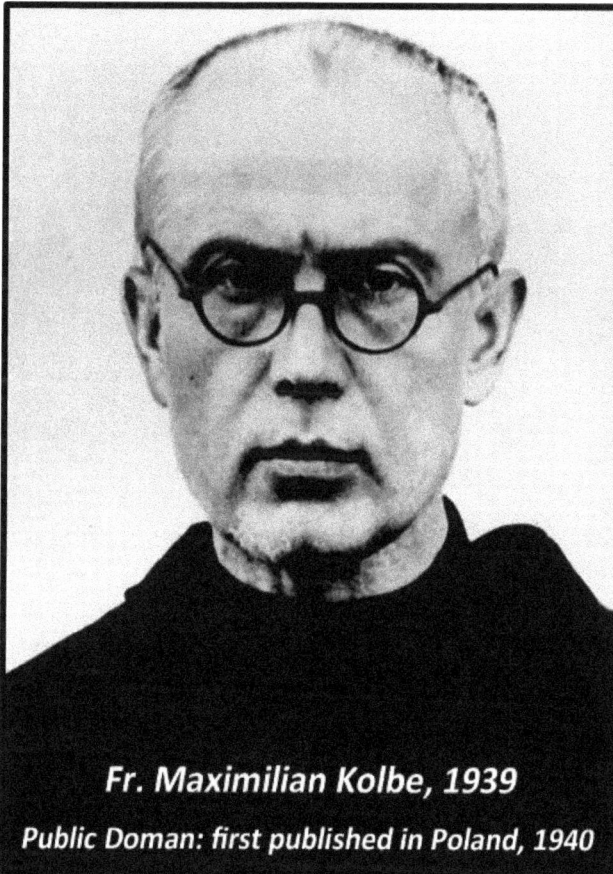

Fr. Maximilian Kolbe, 1939
Public Doman: first published in Poland, 1940

CHAPTER TEN: EPILOGUE

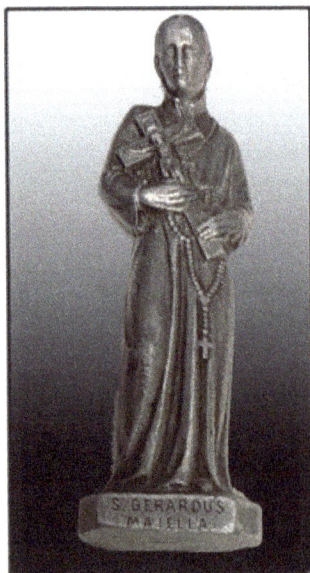

Saint Gerardus Majella is the patron saint of expectant mothers and young children. This is a picture of the small statue given the young boy by his father before he was wheeled into the operating room six weeks after the accident for the cranioplasty to close the hole in his skull. For the six weeks prior to his second operation, the child had not been without his hard-plated Minnesota Twins baseball cap, covering the soft spot in the right side of his head. The only time it had left his head during waking hours was one afternoon at Detroit Lakes, 30 miles east of Moorhead, Minnesota, when he fell off the end of the dock. The hat came floating to the surface, but he did not; at least, not for a few seconds.

I still have the statuette today. It sits on the top shelf of my locker at work. I still remember the first day I held it in my hand…When I was 4-years-old, St. Gerardus filled my palm completely; and I remember the weight of it pushing my hand down to the sheet, and I remember the warmth it had absorbed from my father's hand before he gave it to me. I remember the nurse wheeling me away through the double doors through which I could see my parents waving, framed by the small glass squares of the twin windows receding.

I kept the statuette in a small wooden box with other treasures for years, then I lost track of it, in some box during some move somewhere in the process of growing up and life happening. Twenty years ago, I was reviewing a record in my office and I asked my nurse to send for the old records from another institution. Remember, this was a decade before the Electronic Medical Record was even a gleam in the administrator's eye.

Suddenly, I had a thought, "Tree, please request my old records from The Neuropsychiatric Institute in Fargo, North Dakota from 1966," I asked, thinking *what are the odds*. Two weeks later, I had a half-inch thick envelope on my desk, but it was a busy day and I tossed it in a seldom used drawer in the desk behind me. I forgot about it. Another decade passed. One morning, I was looking for some mundane object in the top drawer to the left of the sink on my side of the bathroom. I can't remember what I was searching for, but in the far back darkness my fingers closed on a familiar object that I hadn't seen for over 30 years. I immediately thought of my old records. I knew exactly where they were.

At the end of the day of clinic, alone in my office, I started on the first page. The note from the emergency room, the x-ray report, the labs, the op-report, progress notes, the cranioplasty; all original documents, a combination of handwritten notes and typed, the rough texture of a typeface font, driven into the paper by miniature metal letters on long, thin arms, palpable against my fingertips. As I read the record, I was gradually overcome by the impossibility of my own existence as I knew it. I had been told my entire life that I was a miracle, but that became only a word to me, ascribed to a head injury most remarkable for the horseshoe shaped scar in my scalp that I had only appreciated for the first time during boot-camp for the ND Army National Guard at the age of 21.

"What the hell is that, soldier?" I remember the drill sergeant asking me at the reception station, where new recruits got their uniforms, shots, and haircuts before moving out to the training units.

"Scalp laceration. SERGEANT!"

"Scalp laceration? PRIVATE!" He screams in my face. "It doesn't look like a scalp laceration to me. You know what it looks like to me? It looks damn purposeful to me. It looks to me like you had an operation. You looks like that guy in that ape movie who had a lobotomy," he says, referencing Charlton Heston in *Planet of the Apes*, which I remembered well, especially the scene at the end when Charlton Heston walks out on the beach in New York and finds the Statue of Liberty sticking out of the stand. He falls to his knees, in profile, his lobotomy scar in sharp relief from the high sun overhead.

"Did you have a lobotomy? PRIVATE!" His voice pulls me back from my reverie. I feel the mist from his bellowing on my face. He knows I feel it too. It's what I call *purposeful*. He comes up to my chin, so he's looking up at me, about four inches from my face, a small-statured Puerto Rican with halitosis, or possibly just onions on a sandwich for lunch.

"I did not have a lobotomy. SERGEANT!" I said, making especially sure to scream out an especially loud *SERGEANT!* at the end, the way they all like it.

"Well you sure act like you've had a lobotomy, PRIVATE!" And then he's gone.

That was a lifetime ago. I remember telling the recruiter at the MEPP station (Military Entrance Processing Point) that I had a head injury and a scalp laceration when I was a young boy, knowing that it was a bit stretching of the truth, but I really had no idea how much of a stretch it was. I only knew that I couldn't complain a few weeks later, after leaving the reception station, in the arid hills of Ft. Leonard Wood when the leather strap of my steel pot, rubbing against the back edge of the plastic plate molded into place 17 years earlier by Dr. Christoferson, precipitated an ulcer. I wrapped some strips of cloth around the headband on either side of the sore and got used to it.

I remember being told about the blood vessels growing before the doctor's eyes. It was part of the miracle story, but as a child the impact wore off with each retelling, and then, in medical school, I figured that it was simply good collateral circulation. There's actually a name for that--the circle of Willis, a circular arrangement of the blood vessels at the base of the brain where each side is connected to the other in the middle, which allows blood to flow from one side to the other. I just had a good circle of Willis I figured. I was wrong. It was much more than that.

I had not the faintest idea of the severity of my injury, my sleep-deprivation-induced CT scan yet two years in the future. It was a quiet afternoon, all the staff gone except my office nurse, Tree, on the other side of the building, always the last to leave. The sun, low in the sky, came in the window, illuminating the King Helmet Tiger Stripe Conch shell I brought up from the bottom of the ocean in Belize when I was 16, holding my breath, the billowing sand forming a cloud in my face as I pulled it free. Behind my left shoulder, on the wall, a portrait of my family on the shore of Lake Michigan, frozen in silent repose. In the top-right drawer of my desk lay the cards and letters of patients that I had treated over the years, patients whose lives I had significantly impacted, in some cases lives that I had saved.

As I read Dr. Christoferson's operative report from that day, the day I should have died, my fingers feeling the subtle texture of the letters like I was reading Braille, I understood the divinity of each subsequent day of the ensuing 50 years. I was overwhelmed by the generosity of the gift my life was, a divine gift that I was heretofore unaware of. I finally realized, after an entire lifetime, it really was a miracle. That much I knew to be true. The dancing dust motes in the sun's light before my eyes turned to a hazy golden glow as I began to cry, the records stretched out before me on my desk, documents all signed by a man whose name began with Christ.

<u>PROGRESS REPORT</u>

July 11, 1968

MELARVIE, Shawn
Case No: #106,799

This boy's parents bring him back for a recheck examination of his plate today. His plate is very well seated, it is very solid, much of the roughness has disappeared as the bone has overgrown the plate somewhat and smoothed out the roughened edges.

I advised the mother that when this boy is nine years old, he should again be psychologically tested but that I really didn't see any need for any further studies or examinations at this time and that if she would get in touch with me when he was nine, I would arrange with Doctor Noble to have him retested at that time but in the meantime I thought he should try to live as completely a normal life as possible.

LEE A. CHRISTOFERSON, M.D.

LAC:jmh

Intro to the Appendices

These are not your grandmother's appendices. Do not overlook them. If I were Elon Musk and this manual my SpaceX, these appendices would be my launching pad, *for you*.

The information is not new, perhaps mildly restated, but the value in them is the checklist format of the things you need to do, in the proper order, and summations of all the strategies so that you can easily find them and refer to them when needed without having to page back through the book.

By this time, you should have read the entire manual. You know what to do, why you should do it, and how. Now, you just need to do it, and that is what these appendices are for.

I wish for you that this be a significant moment, this moment of change. I hope that you have changed your thoughts about your diet and the energy of food, because if you have, all this is permanent. It is forever. It is like you go to bed one night and the sky is blue, and when you wake up, the sky is orange.

Your world has changed. A mental gear in your brain has clicked into place. You can't go back to the world that was before because that would be irrational; it would be crazy, and that, you are not. You are most sane, and you know exactly what you should do. This is your checklist. 5…4…3…2…1…Ready to Launch!

I bet you never read a book with four endings. I love endings because that means a new beginning. Best wishes. God Bless.

APPENDICES

APPENDIX A: HOW TO START

I am hoping that you have completed the diet manual because then you know how important it is to establish a starting point. It is a momentous moment for you. It will separate the time that was before from the time that came after, because this will be forever. There is no reason to go back after knowing what you now know. This is not a simple diet plan you are following. This is a new way of thinking. You are changing your thoughts, and you know what that means.

Please do two things.

1. Record your measurements in the chart below in ink. The beginning column is the most important. You may take measurements monthly, but the first column is the MOST important—the beginning. Most likely you wouldn't need a full year. If you use a phone app or a program on your computer, that's OK too, but write it down here first so it is done rather than something you'll *get around to*.

	Beginning	1	2	3	4	5	6	7	8	9	10	11	12
DATE													
Weight													
BMI													
Measurments													
Neck														
Chest														
Waist														
Hips														

2. Write a short note of encouragement and support to your future self. Write why you're doing this and write something meaningful to you. Something short, that fits on this page. What is your GOAL?

_____
_____
_____
_____
_____

APPENDIX B: HOW TO PREPARE YOUR CASTLE

Your home must be safe. If you live alone or with a spouse or significant other also on a diet, this will be easier. If not, and you are living with other non-dieters, it will take a little more work.

First, let's address the former: everyone is changing their world. You must throw away all the bad stuff. Get the garbage can from the garage, the one with the damp and mold in the bottom from all that nasty trash, and put it on a rug in the kitchen.

Open everything from the lists below and dump it into the trash. This is kind of like those scenes in the movies where the alcoholic is dumping liquor down the drain and you're watching and thinking to yourself *yeah, finally, all right, time to get on with things and a happy ending*. This time though, it's you in the movie and it's your happy ending. Dumping the poison, opened, into the nasty trash prevents you from a possible moment of weakness an hour later. No way, you think. Don't be too sure. Don't take any chances and run the risk of a humiliating experience.

From the fridge/freezer, throw these away:
1. Ice cream and any frozen desserts
2. French fries
3. Frozen pizza, bread dough or equivalents (pasta)
4. Frozen fruits *that are not whole or unsweetened.* Beware "healthy" fruit bases and mixes, check label for added sugars, flavoring, and other unnatural additives.
5. Frozen TV dinners unless specifically lean/low-calorie/low carb. In general, it is best to eat fresh foods, but if you're in a rush...
6. Frozen waffles, pancakes
7. Frozen veggie-burgers that are higher-carb and lower-protein
8. Heavily breaded frozen entrées
9. Pretzels, onion rings, pizza rolls, etc.
10. Yogurt: be careful, even probiotic yogurts can have a lot of sugar.
11. Fruit juice concentrates
12. Frozen whipped topping: corn syrup, bad fats
13. ANYTHING else that has 2x more carbs than protein, added sugars, high-fructose corn syrup; or, if it causes your Spidey-sense to tingle.

From the cupboards and pantry, take these things, open them and dump them down your figurative drain. By now, the frozen foods are melting, and all will be beyond salvage.

1. All chips, even the lower-fat ones. I'm not saying you'll never have another chip, you may, on occasion, at a summer picnic or at someone's house, but not in your castle during the beginning days.
2. White bread, white pasta, rolls, buns, bagels, muffins
3. Pretzels, crackers (unless multi-grain, whole wheat)
4. Non-ketogenic, non-whole wheat, high-protein pancake/waffle mixes
5. White rice cakes
6. Canned baked beans, canned fruits in sugar or with added sugar
7. Any vegetables or fruits that come in bags as chips; they might sound healthy, but they are fried typically and have added preservatives. They definitely are too far removed from being recently pulled from the ground.
8. Colored pasta, which implies is from a vegetable; there's not enough vegetable in it to make a difference.
9. Colored wraps for sandwiches (see #8), or other wraps, other than high-protein, whole wheat, lower carb, which may be ok.
10. Noodle soup kits
11. Reduced fat anything (peanut butter, mayonnaise); reduced fat equals more sugar, high fructose corn syrup.
12. Most dry cereals: especially the flavored ones the kids like, but all are suspect. Read the labels for added sugars, total carbs, protein, fat.
13. Flavored instant cereals, like oatmeal; the added sugars aren't worth it.
14. Whole wheat breads or crackers that DO NOT have "whole grains" on the ingredient label. It may say so on the front, but if the first flour listed in the small print is *enriched wheat flour* or *unbleached,* it is not whole grain.
15. Energy, diet or nutty healthy-looking bars that have 0 fiber, minimal protein or much more than twice as much carbs as protein.
16. Commercial salad dressings: high in sodium and sugar and fat; but mainly, the serving size is small, and you probably use at least two.
17. Powdered coffee creamer has trans-fat, artificial flavors, added sugars.
18. Anything that says "100 Calories" or less is probably bad. It may only be 100 calories, but most likely it is 100 bad calories. Read the label.

19. Pop Tarts or equivalent
20. Dried fruit has a lot of sugar and is very dense and easy to eat too much of.
21. Bottled teas, soda, energy drinks: these have incredible amounts of sugars no matter what other "healthy stuff" they have. Even diet drinks should be avoided.
22. Yogurt covered stuff: tastes great, less filling, and lots of sugar.
23. ANYTHING else that has 2x more carbs than protein, added sugars, high-fructose corn syrup; or if it causes your Spidey-sense to tingle.

Now. *What do you do if you are an Army-of-One on a diet?*

Ideally, you would do the same thing because eating well and healthy is the right way for everyone to eat, but let's say you have some pushback. In that case, throw all the things away from the above lists that your family or non-dieting spouse can live without. It is likely that many of the things are your past preferences and may be specific to you.

For those things your spouse or family must have, segregate them in separate spaces; a different cupboard or a different shelf in the pantry or the fridge or freezer. You will be cleaning house, so there should be plenty of space left for all that categorization, and also for the next part (Append. C), but first, a word of caution.

Many foods, perishable and non, are packaged to look and sound healthy. If they say low-fat, low-calorie or wheat, they should be immediately suspect. Foods that are packaged for a shelf-life often require preservatives, are high-sodium and have additives that are not great. Make sure you read the label for the things I mentioned above, more often than not, you will put the item back on the shelf.

APPENDIX C: HOW TO EAT IN YOUR CASTLE

I do not have the time or the space for a cookbook. That is not my objective. As I stated previously, in Phase I, please pick a cookbook of the diet plan you think would be the easiest, like the Mediterranean Diet. Make sure it says quick and easy, or similar language on the front. You can also search for recipes online for what you would like to prepare. Use search words like low carb, healthy, keto, associated with the food, *for example keto chicken recipes*. However, this requires time and when you start it is better to have more of a plan in mind, even if it's 2-3 quick easy meals repeated over the course of a week or two, until you get your sea legs.

We still need food in our castle, so let us continue.

Things you can put in your freezer/fridge.
1. Whole fruit: (I like blueberries) w/o added sugar, should have 3-4 grams of fiber/serving, and will have about 3x as many carbs as fiber.
2. All frozen vegetables: most don't have added sugar but check anyway.
3. Unsalted nuts: almonds, pecans, walnuts; these things are high in fat, even if good, and shouldn't be a *frequent* snack of significance.
4. Edamame is a high-protein, no sugar, high-fiber soybean snack or side that is quick and easy in the microwave, you sprinkle sea-salt over it.
5. Frozen squash, like butternut: no added sugar and is a great side or in stir-fry or blended into a soup.
6. Frozen avocado chunks: can be handy in the Northwoods when fresh not available.
7. Fish, chicken, bison, grass-fed beef or lean beef, grass-fed sausages or chicken sausage: sausage is processed and higher in sodium and should be not a routine dish, maybe once a week.
8. Greek yogurt without added sugar
9. Cottage cheese; Hard cheese
10. Olives
11. Almond milk: we use this in our shakes.
12. Organic milk is generally higher in omega-3 fatty acids and cows are not given antibiotics.
13. Fresh vegetables: our staples are red and white onions, mushrooms, spinach or power greens or mixed salad greens; sometimes bok-choy.
14. Limes, lemons, apples, pears, peaches (I don't routinely have fruit).

Things you can put in your cupboards and pantry.
1. Fresh vegetables on the counter: squash, sweet potatoes, avocados
2. Low sodium chicken and beef broth in cans or cartons
3. Canned goods: tomatoes, mushrooms, tuna, chicken, sardines, clams (clam chowder), beans w/o added sugars (no baked beans).
4. Chia seeds: we add this to our shakes, good source of good fat and fiber, a superfood they say.
5. Hemp seed: we put this over our salads.
6. Salad topping
7. Cauliflower rice
8. Kodiak Power cakes or equivalent: high-protein, lower-carb waffle/pancake mix
9. Steel cut oats: not too often as is higher carb than other options.
10. Whole grain crackers: these are all rather similar in that they are approximately 15-20 net carbs per serving of 12-15 crackers (small ones). At least they do have fiber and protein but pay attention to the serving size and do not eat out of the box, put a serving in a small dish, and it will be small.
11. Coconut oil powders, acacia powder, and similar that can be added to blended shakes.

Flavoring, seasoning, oils to have in your castle. All the above is fine and well, but you still need the other things, like:
1. Olive oils: extra virgin is good for pan frying; flavored olive oils are popular, like dill, garlic, and can be used for salads or frying protein entrees like fish or chicken.
2. Avocado oil is another oil that is good for cooking.
3. Vinegar, wine vinegar, balsamic: oil and vinegar is a much better salad dressing than the commercially prepared; you can add a salad topping to take it up a notch or even make fresh guacamole (red onion, olive oil, lime, avocado, cilantro).
4. Salt, pepper, other seasonings: great sources of flavor and no calories
5. Soy sauce, brown mustard, garlic, etc.

*Intermittent Fasting is not a requirement, but it is a powerful option. At the minimum, I would implement a 12-hour fast, which is simply *not eating after dinner*. The next advancement would be an 18-hour fast, which would be skipping breakfast as well and eating between 12 and 6 p.m., or some variation thereof.

Meals to eat in your castle.
OK. You now have a castle full of good calories to fill that fuel cell in your belly. *What now?*

Just to make this easy, let me game out a few meals for you if you don't have your cookbook yet. These are things that I do. It is simply a matter of reading labels. You will find the things you prefer.

Breakfast:
Super easy if you're fasting:
Large glass of water with Benefiber and/or a couple of fiber gummies, coffee with cream or a coconut oil creamer (my favorite). I know that sweetener is bad, but I can't drink coffee without a little of it. Maybe I'll grow up some day.

If you're not fasting:
1. Eggs and vegetables, mushrooms, and a link of chicken sausage, if you must.
2. Once or twice a week: Hi-protein, lower-carb waffles, sugar-free syrup.
3. Greek yogurt and a grapefruit or equivalent.

Lunch:
1. A shake with almond milk, frozen blueberries, chia seeds (2 tsp), acacia powder (1-2 tsp), Greek yogurt, two packs of sweetener (I'm sorry. I am intermittently weak).
2. Sardines and 12 whole-wheat crackers, hard cheese
3. Tuna, vegetables
4. True whole-grain crackers, bread or wraps 2-3x/wk.
5. Deli meat is OK, but shouldn't be a regular staple because it is processed and usually higher in sodium, but it is low carb.
6. Salad with a protein topping of choice

One last idea: mail order protein entrées. We've been ordering a box of frozen seafood once a month from *Great Alaska Seafood*. We get different cuts of fish that are all individually wrapped in appropriate portion sizes. It arrives packed in dry ice and is very good. They came with suggested recipes, one being a cream sauce that I use most of the time. We cook and eat dinner in about 30 minutes: fish entrée, frozen vegetables, sweet potato or squash, salad with topping and sometimes guacamole.

Dinner:
1. Entrée: Beef, chicken or fish from your freezer; the beef or chicken can be sliced into strips for a stir-fry, or can be grilled and can have steamed vegetables as a side, or a salad with oil and vinegar and a salad topping and/or guacamole; can have a sweet potato or squash as a side dish or a whole-grain rice or equivalent.
2. Other sides: cauliflower rice, zucchini noodles (can make these with a simple hand-held noodle blade).
3. True "whole grain" pasta, not whole wheat is ok periodically, if it's ground, it's no good from our standpoint. This might be hard to find. In general, try to avoid grain, but if you need a break...
4. Explore creative keto-recipes online, like cabbage lasagna. There are many.
5. Chili is easy: ground meat, legumes, vegetables, anything else you like; put Greek yogurt or sour cream on top; make 2-3 nights worth, repeat.

Dessert:
1. Should be infrequent because if you eat a lower carbohydrate diet that is more generous in good fats, the higher fats will cause you to feel fuller sooner. Many times, you may eat too fast, and your satiety doesn't have a chance to catch up, so try to eat slower and if you feel like you need something else, wait 10 minutes. Fresh fruit is fine, maybe a smaller shake, and rarely, you might make a keto-dessert, but you shouldn't get into the habit of having a dessert every night. You don't need it.
2. There will be enough times that you will be eating out with friends or as a guest and the opportunity for a real dessert will present itself, and you will partake because it is rather rare, and as I have said, our diet is not a religion. We will not go to hell if we break our fast or have a dessert. The rule is that dessert is sensible and seldom.

One last thing: The odds are in your favor. The market forces have demanded accountability in some measure. All packaged foods are labeled, even if deceptively at times; still, low-carb, gluten-free, high-protein, no trans-fats are labels rarely seen 10 years ago that are now ubiquitous.

Now. Take the garbage can back out of the kitchen and go shopping for good fuel to stock your castle with.

APPENDIX D: HOW TO EAT OUTSIDE THE WALL

This is difficult because it is common, and restaurants, especially fast-food chains, do not make it easy. By now, you already know enough to make the proper choices, but I will make some general suggestions below.

1. Fast food burger joint: For me, this would be hard, because I really like burgers and French fries and chips, so it would be hard for me to order the sensible items, which are grilled chicken salad (better, because no bread) or grilled chicken sandwich; but, that usually comes with fries which are bad, as can be the high-fat sandwich spread. Some of the breakfast options are ok, like an egg sandwich with a slice of ham.
2. Fast food subway place: Easier, because no fries and have to pay extra for chips. It's best if the whole wheat is whole grain, like the 9-grain wheat or honey oat bread from Subway.
3. Steak place: Even easier for a dinner; can decline the bread, which I usually can't do, but it's less than once a week. You can pick a leaner cut of beef, or poultry or fish. I like the New York Strip or flank or flatiron. Ribeye and prime rib are fattier and have more calories.
   You get two sides; order the salad that has fewer calories and the vegetable, or what my wife and I do is one of us orders the sweet potato and the other orders the vegetable, and we split them.

Restaurants that are centered around pasta and bread will be difficult. Mexican restaurants are also difficult because of the chips (bad) and salsa.

As previously stated, the odds are in your favor. Everything on the menus are labeled for the most part, at least in the major chains, and most every restaurant has a small section of the menu more specific to proper choices. Whether or not you can restrict your selection to that smaller part remains to be seen; however, by avoiding breading, choosing leaner cuts of protein, and choosing vegetable sides or splitting a sweet potato rather than a white potato are all things you can do.

Ideally, eating outside the wall will be infrequent. Developing a pattern of behavior of quick easy meal preparation for one meal a day (dinner) is preferable.

APPENDIX E: THE SEVEN BIOLOGICAL TRUTHS

1. **INSULIN TURNS OFF FAT METABOLISM AND STORES ENERGY (FOOD) AS FAT OR GLYCOGEN.**

2. **CARBOHYDRATE/SUGAR IS THE PRIMARY MACRONUTRIENT THAT CAUSES THE RELEASE OF INSULIN.**

3. **PROTEIN ALSO CAUSES THE RELEASE OF INSULIN, NOT AS MUCH AS CARBOHYDRATE, BUT IT STILL DOES.**

4. **FAT IS STORED ENERGY. IT DOES NOT CAUSE A SIGNIFICANT RELEASE OF INSULIN IF INGESTED.**

5. **GLYCOGEN IS STORED ENERGY. IT IS THE STORAGE FORM OF CARBOHYDRATE/GLUCOSE.**

6. **INSULIN TURNS NEARLY ALL INGESTED FOOD NOT USED FOR METABOLIC NEEDS INTO GLUCOSE, THEN INTO GLYCOGEN, THEN INTO FAT, IN THAT ORDER.**

7. **YOUR BODY WILL ALWAYS BURN GLUCOSE OR GLYCOGEN FIRST, WHEN GIVEN THE CHOICE.**

If this is all new to you, or if you would find it a helpful behavioral management tool, you could print off this list and tape it to the inside of your cupboard as a reminder.

APPENDIX F: WHAT YOU NEED TO KNOW ABOUT EXERCISE

Unless you are a competitive athlete, the primary purpose of exercise is for **stress reduction** and **sense of well-being**. It also **preserves lean body mass** so that you suffer less from the age-related drop in metabolism and the associated musculoskeletal conditions such as osteoporosis (25) and arthritis, including wedge compressions of the thoracic vertebral bodies. *Remember Quasimodo?*

Types of aerobic exercise:
1. Walking*
2. Rowing*
3. Swimming*
4. Bike riding*; open road or stationary /recumbent
5. Dancing*
6. Jogging/running/treadmill/elliptical trainer
7. Cross country skiing*
8. Aerobic exercise programs on DVD, or at gym; you have a leader to follow, which is motivating and helpful.
9. Jumping rope
10. Fishing: *I'm kidding.*
11. Ice skating*
12. Tennis
13. Basketball; is kind of a combination of aerobic and resistance.

*The * above five are all low impact, unless you are a very aggressive dancer; or, if you aren't paying attention on your bike, skid on some gravel, catapult over a guardrail headfirst still clipped into you bike pedals, then inadvertently do a complete 360 before landing in the shallow creek 12-feet below and breaking only both your legs. That's definitely high impact.*

Aerobic training should be at least twice a week, preferably 3-4x/week; at least 20-30 minutes. It really can't be too much. It should be palatable. It could be riding a stationary bike or walking/jogging on a treadmill during the evening news or football (or something you enjoy watching on TV).

If you are obese or have arthritic issues you should do a low-impact exercise, otherwise, you should check with your health care provider.

If you don't know what to pick, do this: start with walking, it is the most obvious. Download a podcast to listen to, or listen to music, or simply be alone with your thoughts, or visit with a fellow walking companion.

Types of resistance training:
1. Free weights are the classical form,
2. Weight machines, as found in gyms and fitness centers.
3. Resistance bands
4. Kettlebell workout
5. Yoga is not an obvious selection; however, one of the most difficult resistance routines in the rigorous P90x program is the yoga one.
6. Machines that combine legs and arms with resistance, usually a combination of peddling and moving your arms together; but this must be against resistance, or it is more aerobic.
7. Using your own body weight: leg squats, pushups, pull-ups, sit-ups.
8. Cross-Fit is popular and is combination of both aerobic and resistance training.

Resistance training is harder for most people because it's not as accessible, as easy or as convenient as walking. Most of the time it requires equipment, even if minimal. I hesitate to recommend a specific weight program regimen because it is easier to injure yourself with resistance training than it is by walking the dog, especially if you've not habitually done it most of your life.

Even resistance bands can be harmful if you lose control of one end. *Ouch*. I know. Rotator cuff injuries, tennis elbow, strained back are all potential injuries. I know that the majority of my readers will be overweight or obese, and I urge caution; however, resistance training is important, more important than you think.

Please do this if you can: If you have no prior experience, join the YMCA or a local fitness club to get started on a resistance training program. Once you know what to do and how to do it, you may then pursue it on your own.

Your primary care provider should have an access point for you as well in this regard as part of a whole-body health program.

If you can't afford a membership or don't have access through your primary care provider, consider this:

From the list on the previous page, the least expensive is #7, using your own body weight, and probably the safest in regard to the potential for causing self-injury. This can be enhanced by using a kettlebell, which will be additive to your body weight; however, even that requires proper form, so you don't strain your back. Yoga is another type of resistance training that utilizes your own body weight, but this also requires instruction to do it properly. Resistance bands or a set of adjustable dumbbells is easier to start with and less intimidating than a barbell with weights. Weight machines take much of the risk of free weights out of the equation, but you need a weight machine, or access to one.

At FatThief.com I've posted some links to videos that will be instructive; still, I would suggest that you seek further assistance on the front end, until you know how to perform your selected modes of resistance training safely and efficiently. You can learn much from videos, and following along with an online trainer, but you will still most likely not be doing the movements as well as you would with personal assistance.

Expert advice is not as far away as you might think. A son or daughter or nephew or niece, or all of the prior with the prefix of "grand," are all potential sources of help. Do you have a football player, gymnast, soccer star, swimmer, etc. in the family? For any sport, resistance training is an important component and these family members would be able to provide guidance and would happily do so.

Another source of help might be your local high-school weight-training coach. The people who are interested and engaged in physical fitness generally welcome discussing it and sharing their insights and tips and general knowledge. If coach is too busy to offer you his or her time for some brief instruction, I am sure he or she could task a stellar young man or woman to do so.

If you still are struggling with what to do and want to do more than 30-minutes of body-weight exercises twice a week, one idea would be to go to a fitness store to buy a kettlebell or adjustable dumbbell set or similar. At a fitness store, or dedicated fitness department of a larger store, you will more likely encounter a salesperson who can offer some hands-on guidance for the proper use of the equipment purchased.

Remember that with any exercise it is important to warm up both before and after, and when beginning to lift any weights, start with smaller weights and more repetitions until you get your sea legs. I am not trying to turn you into a superhero. Our focus is on losing weight and preserving lean body mass. Do a resistance training workout 2x/week for 20-30 minutes.

As you get faster and stronger, you will progress to heavier weights or longer times and may branch into other forms of resistance training. You might even become a superhero.

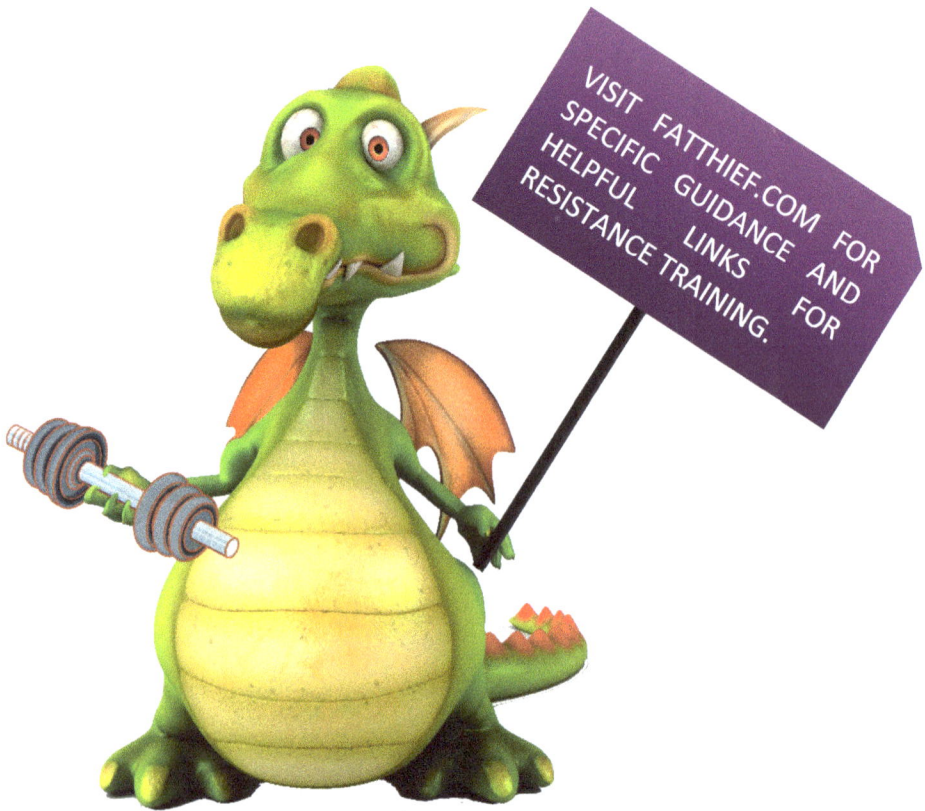

VISIT FATTHIEF.COM FOR SPECIFIC GUIDANCE AND HELPFUL LINKS FOR RESISTANCE TRAINING.

APPENDIX G: THE TEN COMMANDMENTS

These directives represent the four phases described in the first sections of the manual. The progression is from a conventional caloric-controlled strategy towards a ketogenic-type, insulin-controlled strategy. You may progress as rapidly as you wish, however, you should start at #1 on the checklist, because starting at #6 won't be as effective long-term without first accomplishing #'s 1-5.

1. ☐**Pick a diet plan**: My bias is towards a low-carb ketogenic, anti-inflammatory strategy. It is my feeling that these diets are easier to comply with as they are less restrictive than the plant-based, animal-product-avoidance strategy; but, you're the boss. Pick whatever you want.

2. ☐ **Prepare your castle**: Make your home a safe place. It is your fortress of solitude that should be impervious to the dragon. Have a strategy for how you're going to eat when outside the wall.

3. ☐ **Use an online basal caloric need calculator** to figure out how many calories you should consume per day to lose 1-2 pounds per week: If you are on one of the diets towards either extreme of extremely low-fat, plant-based; or, low-carb ketogenic, counting calories is less important, but I think it is still helpful for a few weeks until you have an appreciation of how many calories are in the foods you eat.
    <https://www.niddk.nih.gov/bwp>

4. ☐ **Be accountable**. Be honest. Control what you eat by keeping a food journal or using a phone app. *Visit FatThief.com for suggestions.*

5. ☐ **Understand the effect insulin** has on your fat metabolism: It's bad. Insulin makes fat.

6. ☐ **Limit your carbohydrate**s to less than 100 grams/day: Zero sugar or refined carbohydrates.

7. ☐ **Implement an intermittent fasting strategy**: Alternating days of fasting, or a daily 12-18 hour extended nighttime fast.

8. ☐ **Understand** that the Dragon of Obesity will kill you: You will live less, and you will live less well than you would otherwise.

9. ☐ **Exercise** is good and necessary, but it's not as important as your diet. Do *something*.

10. ☐ **Resistance training** preserves lean muscle mass: Implement a resistance training program so you won't turn into a dorsal-kyphotic Quasimodo.

*A good behavioral activation technique would be to display the list and check the boxes when competed.

APPENDIX H: FREUDIAN PSYCHOANALYTICAL STRATEGIES

You need techniques/thoughts/ideas to control your inner baby. One list won't work for everybody because the most powerful techniques, thoughts, ideas are likely specific to each individual inner baby. This list is only limited by your imagination. Let me get you started. It is important that you identify those techniques specific to you and to add to the list other techniques, thoughts or ideas that are specific to you.

These are *behavioral activation techniques* that may allow you to modify your behavior to a positive end. One of the primary functions of any one of them is to serve as a brake, so you have **time to think**, time for your egos to act.

1. **Stop. Think.** How many calories is one serving? How big is one serving? Am I hungry? Am I angry, sad, bored? Why am I angry/sad/bored? *Is it worth it?*
2. **Have a realistic or idealistic image** of yourself as you would wish to be. This could be a picture from a time before you were overweight or obese if that ever was the case, or an image of another with a body habitus you'd like to achieve. Have it in your mind. You might have it in an inside cupboard at home, or in your wallet or purse or on your phone, but at least have it in your mind. Imagine it. *Is it still worth it?*
3. Think of the ingredients as poison, the combination of bad fats and sugar; the accompanying surge of insulin; the storage of fat, like the glistening translucent whorls cut from a fatty steak being stored in your body.
4. Say a short prayer or a meditation mantra.
5. Pinch your subcutaneous tissue to either side of your belly button. How thick is it? *Is it still worth it?*
6. Close your eyes, blink, turn away, give yourself some positive affirmation. I am loved. I am a good person. I can do this for myself. I choose a different reality. I choose a different universe. *Is it still worth it?*
7. Leave. If you're in the breakroom, take the time to do any of the above or equivalent while you're leaving.
8. If you succumb, all is not lost. Yet. With that first bite of whatever it is, does it taste as good as you imagined it would, or is it stale, rather tasteless? How good is it, really? *Is it still worth it?*
9. *...you are only limited by your imagination. Please add at least two more to the list.*

APPENDIX I: MINDFUL STRATEGIES
The fuller explanations are found beginning on page 132

1. Identify those core beliefs and assumptions that are faulty or distorted. *
2. Start each day with a meditation or prayer.
3. Go to your church or special place regularly.
4. Acquire a talisman:
    a. Piece of jewelry of special meaning
    b. Place inspirational quotes, pictures in places you see every day.
    c. Place motivational quote or picture in the kitchen inside a cupboard door, at your place of employment.
5. Use mental talismans (mantras).
6. Harness the power of a social support network.
7. Start a journal or blog.

These too, are behavioral activation techniques, those things you do so that you modify your behavior to make the good choice rather than the bad. These are a few ways of developing good habits and positive thoughts and actions to replace the bad habits and negative thoughts and actions. This is a list you should be able to add to. Add one or two things of your own, or more. A primary purpose is for these actions and reminders to allow you time to do the right thing, time for your egos to overcome the impulse.

*#1 is the biggest because without addressing that it is unlikely that anything will follow. Remember from page 132: "One such book that has been around for many years and can help you with this is **Mind Over Mood** (19)."

If there is any doubt about the health of your core beliefs, at least start with a self-help book such as the above for further introspection and thought and/or talk to your primary care provider about your concerns, and he or she will refer you on for further help if needed.

Do this: If you are concerned about your core beliefs, talk to your health care provider.

APPENDIX J: SOCIAL SUPPORT IDEAS

Support starts at home. I would hope you have the support of your family at home. This may not be true in every case for whatever reason, in which case it will be more difficult, but there are other avenues of camaraderie and support available for those joined by a common purpose.

The next level of support, outside of the home would be a group of **friends or fellow employees** engaged in a similar effort. There may not be a formal structure, like an email or social platform group, although that is easy enough to do and would be beneficial, but it takes one with the savvy and motivation to do so.

The next level would be a **professional, clinic-based level of support**, which could be rendered by your primary care provider that would involve scheduled visits to the clinic for accountability and counseling, possibly even a referral to Behavioral Management for individual and/or group counseling.

Somewhat like the above would be the **commercial weight-loss programs**, the most well-known being *Weight Watchers* and *Jenny Craig*, which involve personal coaching and periodic accountability measures. The commercial programs have a monthly cost and are interested in selling meal plans, snacks, and possibly supplements and other products.

The next levels of support are the social networking platforms:

1. **Facebook**: You need a FB account of course. Login. In the search bar at the top of the page type in the diet you are following, like "keto," and then click on the "Groups" tab on the tool bar underneath the search bar. All the groups will be displayed. You can type in Mediterranean, Vegetarian, Paleo, anti-inflammatory, anything. Browse and join.

2. **Online forums**:
   a. Obesityhelp.com: a portal that includes forums of common concerns and topics; community access to multiple groups; recipes; resources; and some products.
   b. Myfitnesspal.com: another portal with more of an emphasis on fitness, but also offering a community and an active blog.
   c. 3fatchicks.com: another popular portal with community, informational articles, a forum and recipes.
3. **App-based**:
   a. Myfitnesspal has an app as well.
   b. Fatsecret.com: has mobile apps for your phone and the ability to track calories; has recipes and nutritional information, weight chart journal, and more. It is available for free and has some good reviews.
   c. Noom is a popular app that has a monthly variable cost.
4. **In-person support groups**:
   a. Obesityaction.org (OAC) is a nonprofit portal that has a support tab on the home page which lists support groups available by state, but you have to join OAC (free) to access the information. Much of the support structure is associated with medical clinics and bariatric/surgical services and there *may be* some marketing of supplements, VeryLowCalorieDiets (VLCD) and surgical services.
   b. In most communities, the local newspaper will list support groups in the back pages, such as Overeaters Anonymous.

There is no shortage of social support. It can be anonymous or not. Other travelers on the road you are traveling can be tremendous sources of support for there is much in common, and it is nearly certain that whatever you are experiencing or struggling with is a problem someone else has already solved or conquered.

The only difficulty is that there is so much, almost too much, choice, and that can be challenging.

Do this: If you are a phone person, I'd try the FatSecret app and join a pertinent FB group for starters.

APPENDIX K: ON STARTING A BLOG

Blog is short for we**B log**. Blogs can be fun, therapeutic, a means of communication, a form of expression, and so much more. My idea for you *of a blog* is as more of a tool from the standpoint of therapeutic-*ness* and journaling. It is a medium that is in the cloud, and available to anyone, anytime, anywhere. It doesn't sound very private, I know, but it can be. It can be all those things in the ether, out there, but only you hold the key. Just make sure it's a good key, and that you don't live in China.

It is hard to lose a blog. Your posts are a snapshot of the time at which you wrote a specific entry. Pictures, video, your deepest thoughts, links you found on the web; a true multimedia record. Your blog could be completely in the dark, known only to you, and who you share a post with; or it can be public, and you can keep some posts private or share them with a select audience.

If you don't like this idea or find it intimidating, then at least consider starting a weight loss journal. It will help you organize your thoughts, say things aloud, as it were, and this may help you find some direction at some point in your life when direction is needed.

The following is a list of some of the most popular free blog providers:
1. Wix.com
2. Squarespace.com
3. Wordpress.com
4. Jimdo.com
5. Site123.com

All these free blog services are easy, and template driven. It as simple as following instructions to get started. You should know that with a free service you will not have a unique url (address) it will be something like <your username.wordpress.com> or similar rather than something cool, like *SoLovedTheWorld.com* or *FatThief.com*.

APPENDIX L: MANTRA IDEAS

The use of mantras is very old and used as a tool to aid in meditation. It is a word or short phrase of meaning that is repeated over and over. It works better if the phrase or sound consists of the long vowel sounds, ending in the consonants that your feel in the chest, like "M" or "N."

There are the traditional Sanskrit mantras, such as "**AUM**" or "Om." It is a sacred sound of Hindu. It translates as *It is, Will Be, or To Become*.

Another from Tibet, "**OM MANI PADME HUM**." It translates approximately as "Hail the Jewel in the Lotus," the jewel being the Buddha.

The English translation from the Torah when God answered Moses, "**I AM THAT I AM**," is yet another.

The mantras from page 133:
"Love is the only miracle there is." *Osho*
"Be the change you wish to see in the world." *Gandi*
"Every day in every way I am getting better and better." *Laura Silva*
"I change my thoughts, I change my world." *Norman Vincent Peale*

The mantra can also offer a pause. It is also a behavioral activation. It is something you can do if placed under stress or your mind draws a blank. You don't know what to do: You almost got killed by a drunk-driver and your heart is racing; someone close to you died--*I am that I am, I am that I am, I am that I am...*
Love is the only miracle there is, love is the only miracle there is...

A mantra can be anything of course. It can be the line of a prayer, *Hail Mary Full of Grace*; a verse of poetry, *Beauty is Truth, and Truth Beauty...A glooming peace this morning with it brings...*Ok, maybe not the last one. A mantra should be a positive aspiration, not the last line from *Romeo and Juliet*.

There are online options to craft a personal mantra if you're interested. Search for *how to create a personalized mantra* and surf away.
Me? I default to *Hail Mary Full of Grace*... One of these days I'll research meditation a bit more.

APPENDIX M: SPIRITUAL STRATEGIES

1. Begin each day with a prayer.
2. End each day with a prayer or work your way through the bible or a book of meditations, or spiritual reading.
3. When you are presented with a choice for which you know the right answer but are struggling with, say a familiar formulaic prayer, like the Our Father or Hail Mary or Act of Contrition or Serenity Prayer.
4. Use a religious talisman, a medallion, ring, bracelet as a source of comfort and strength as a reminder of your commitment. Feel it. See it. Remember why it is special to you.
5. Use a religious mantra, a favorite passage from the bible, like:
   a. Jesus, pray for me.
   b. Lord, have mercy.
   c. Yaweh.
   d. Lord Jesus, help me.
   e. I can do all things through Christ who strengthens me.
   f. This is the day the Lord has made.
6. Display reminders of your Faith and Commitment.
   a. Place these where you see them daily, at home when getting ready for the day or ending the day; at work; in your car.
   b. They can be quotes, pictures, medals, statues, a cross, an icon.
7. Once a week, do something bigger.
   a. Go to church or quiet place associated with your faith.
   b. Be still. Use your mantra, think of the things that need thinking of, important things, like your faults, your graces, how you've treated others the week past, what you could have done better.
   c. Record your thoughts and progress in a spiritual journal.

WORKS CITED

1. **Guyton, Arthur C.** Chapters: 67,68,69,78. [book auth.] Arthur c Guyton. *Textbook of Medical Physiology.* Philadelphia : W.B Saunders Company, 1986, pp. 808-834, 923-936.

2. *The acute effect of fat on insulin secretion.* **Collier, G R, et al.** 2, February 1988, Journal of Clinical Endocrinoglogy and Metabolism, Vol. 66, pp. 323-326.

3. **Smithsonian.** Human Origins. *Smithsonian National Museum of Natural History.* [Online] August 24, 2018. [Cited: July 17, 2019.] http://humanorigins.si.edu/evidence/human-fossils/species/ardipithecus-kadabba.

4. *Basics in clinical nutrition: Simple and stress starvation.* **K, Bareendregt, et al.** 2008, European e-Journal of Clinical Nutrition and Metabolism (2008) 3, Vol. 3, pp. e267-e271.

5. *Effects of low (LCD) and VLCD (VLCD) energy diets on metabolic rate and body composition in obese (fa/fa) Zucker rats.* **MJ, Stock.** 1989; 13 Suppl 2, International Journal of Obesity, pp. 61-65.

6. **WD, McArdle, FI, Katch and VL, Katch.** Exercise Physiology: Ch 9. *Exercise Physiology: Energy, Nutrition & Human Performance; Sixth Edition.* Baltimore : Lippincott, Williams & Wilkins, 2007, pp. 200-201.

7. *Features of a successful therapeutic fast of 382 days' duration.* **WK, Stewart and LW, Fleming.** 1973, Postgraduate Medical Journal (March 1973) 49, 203-209, pp. 203-209.

8. *Chronic Inflammation in Obesity and the Metabolic Syndrome.* **R, Monteiro and I, Azevedo.** Article ID 289645, 10 pages, Porto, Portugal : Hindawi Publishing Corporation, 2010, Mediators of Inflammation, Vol. 2010.

9. **CDC.** Centers for Disease Control and Prevention. *CDC 24/7: Saving Lives, Protecting People.* [Online] May 15, 2015. [Cited: July 17, 2019.] https://www.cdc.gov/healthyweight/effects/index.html.

10. *Age-related and disease-related muscle loss: the effect of diabetes, obesity, and other diseases.* **Kalyani, RR, M, Corriere and L, Ferrucci.** 10, October 2014, Lancet Diabetes Endocrinology, Vol. 2, pp. 819-829.

11. *Effects of Exercise and Physical Activity on Anxiety.* **Anderson, Elizabeth and Shivakumar, Geetha.** 27, April 23, 2013, Frontiers in Psychiatry, Vol. 4.

12. *Resting metabolic rate of obese patients under very low calorie ketogenic diet.* **D, Gomez-Arbelaez, et al.** Feb 17, 2018; 15:18, Nutrition & Metabolism.

13. *Diet Soda Intake and Risk of Incident Metabolic Syndrome and Type 2 Diabetes in the Multi-Ethnic Study of Atherosclerosis (MESA).* **JA, Nettleton, et al.** 4, April 2009, Diabetes Care, Vol. 32, pp. 688-694.

14. *Hypothyroidism and obesity: An intriguing link.* **Sanyal, Debmalya and Raychaudhum, Moutusi.** July-August 2016, Indian Journal of Endocrinology and Metabolism, pp. 554-557.

15. *The Genetics of Obesity.* **Herrera, Blanca M and Lingren, Cecilia M.** 6, December 2010, Current Diabetes Reports, Vol. 10, pp. 498-505.

16. **Futurism.** The Many Worlds Interpretation or the Copenhagen Interpretation. *Futurism/The Byte.* [Online] July 14, 2014. [Cited: July 18, 2019.] https://futurism.com/the-many-world-interpretation-or-the-copenhagen-interpretation.

17. **S, McLeod.** Id, Ego and Superego. *Simply Psychology.* [Online] Feb 5, 2016. https://www.simplypsychology.org/psyche.html.

18. *Sugar Addiction: From Evolution to Revolution.* **D, Wiss, N, Avena and P, Rada.** 545, November 7, 2018, Frontiers in Psychiatry, Vol. 9.

19. **D, Greenberger and C, Padesky.** *Mind Over Mood.* 2nd. s.l. : The Guilford Press, 2015.

20. **O, Schroeder Michael.** Behavioral Activation: the Depression Therapy You've Likely Never Heard Of. *US News.* [Online] November 24, 2016. https://health.usnews.com/wellness/mind/articles/2016-11-24/behavioral-activation-the-depression-therapy-youve-likely-never-heard-of.

21. *Obesity with Comorbid Eating Disorders: Associated health Risks and Treatment Approaches.* **Q, Luz Felipe, et al.** 7, June 25, 2018, Nutrients, Vol. 10.

22. *The relationship between body mass index, binge eating disorder and suicidality.* **Brown, Krystal Lyn B, LaRose, Jessica G and Mezuk, Briana.** 196, Richmond : s.n., June 15, 2018, BMC Psychiatry, Vol. 18.

23. *Called to Evangelize: The Story of Adele Brise and the Mariophany that Changed her Life.* **Looney, Edward.** Article 10, 2011, Marian Studies, Vol. 62.

24. **Franciscan Media.** Saint Maximilian Mary Kolbe. *Franciscan Media.* [Online] 2019. https://www.franciscanmedia.org/saint-maximilian-mary-kolbe/.

25. *The effects of progresive resistance training on bone density: a review.* **Layne Jennifer E., M.S. and E., Nelson Miriam.** 1, January 31, 1999, Med Science Sports Exercise, Vol. 31, pp. 25-30.

26. *A Historical and Theoretical Review of Cognitive Behavioral Therapies: From Structural Self-Knowledge to Functional Processes.* **M, Ruggiero Giovanni, et al.** 4, April 13, 2018, Journal of Rational Emotive Cognitive Behavioral Therapy, Vol. 36, pp. 378-403.

27. **Alcoholics Anonymous World Services, Inc.** The Twelve Steps of Alcoholics Anonymous. *Alcoholics Anonymous.* [Online] 8 2016. [Cited: July 18, 2019.] https://www.aa.org/assets/en_US/smf-121_en.pdf.

28. **Catholic Online.** St. Gerard Majella. *Catholic Online.* [Online] [Cited: July 18, 2019.] https://www.catholic.org/saints/saint.php?saint_id=150.

29. **Kelly, Brian.** First Approved Marian Apparition in the US, Champion, Wisconsin. *Catholocism.org.* [Online] December 23, 2010. https://catholicism.org/first-approved-marian-apparition-in-the-us-champion-wisconsin.html.

ACKNOWLEDGMENTS

When I reached the end of my first draft, I knew that it was only the beginning. By the end of my eighth version I felt I was ready to share it with my brother-in-law, Clem Gerhardt. I knew him as an intelligent, avid reader and I trusted that he would give me his honest opinion, and I was not disappointed. It was Clem's input that was the impetus for the most dramatic change in my manuscript and global approach to the problem of obesity for the reader and for that I am eternally grateful.

There is only one reader who suffered all versions of the manuscript and that of course is my wife, Susan, much of the time being read a lengthy passage in broken sentences as I edited in real time. She also was my initial filter for the many graphics and told me if something was funny, or not, and much of the humor in the finished graphics are secondary to her input. She has been a lifelong source of support in all my efforts without which I would have accomplished little, and this most recent effort is no exception.

Although an English Lit. major, that pleasant experience was remote enough such that the heavy burden of corrective action with a red pen fell to Jen Zettel-Vandenhouten. I am not sure how many pens she went through, not sure I want to know, but I am so very grateful for her kind guidance and gentle treatment of "my child." Only she will know the true frailty of my grasp of the English language, or at least, punctuation.

Ruth Brendemuehl was kind, tolerant and generous with her time to bring the characters of my graphics to life, drawing what I needed, doing what I could not do myself. Thank you, Ruth.

Perhaps my fiercest critic to my face was my good friend and colleague, Dr. Martin Finck. Martin didn't read the book, rather, he rejected 18 book covers and at least as many titles. I was ready to pull the trigger on most of them and always found enough people to say that they liked this one or that one to assuage my conviction, but not Martin, who is quite comfortable with criticism, and for that valuable quality of his I am thankful. I am also appreciative of the surgical staff for their input and my fellow employees at Door County Medical Center who shared their input with me over the course of the past year.

My good friend, Don Renfrew was the last one to read my book, which was a good thing because he found subtle errors that I had trouble seeing even after he told me where they were. Of course, he's an excellent radiologist with a great intellect, and finding small things in a sea of images, as he does every day, well suits him for this particular task. My absolute last reader, Judi Sowl, RDN, CD found two errors that escaped the expert eye of Dr. Renfrew. Me thinks she would have made an excellent radiologist; however, she is already an excellent nutritionist.

Lastly, an honorable mention of *Charles Dickens* and *John Keats* is in order; the former for a shamelessly paraphrased sentence, the last sentence of a *Tale of Two Cities*, one of my favorites, and the latter for the use of a fragment of a poem, both instances quite towards the end. If you know of them, you will recognize them, if you don't, you are free to think me clever, if for no other reason than the use thereof.

ABOUT THE AUTHOR

Shaun Melarvie, MD, is a general surgeon in Northeastern Wisconsin on the shores of Lake Michigan, North of Lambeau Field some fifty miles. He graduated from the University of North Dakota, summa cum laude, with a B.A. in English Literature and minors in biology and chemistry, and four years later from the UND School of Medicine. He completed a general surgery residency at the University of Nebraska before moving to his rural practice in Wisconsin.

www.ingramcontent.com/pod-product-compliance
Lightning Source LLC
Chambersburg PA
CBHW061226270326
41928CB00024B/3341